Insulin Pumps
and Continuous
Glucose Monitoring
Made Easy

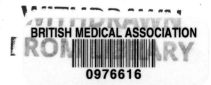

Insulin Pumps and Continuous Glucose Monitoring
Made Easy

Sufyan Hussain MA MB BChir MRCP PhD

Honorary Clinical Lecturer,
Imperial College London;
Specialist Registrar in Diabetes, and Endocrinology,
Imperial College Healthcare NHS Trust,
London UK

Nick Oliver BSc MBBS FRCP

Reader in Diabetes,
Imperial College London;
Consultant in Diabetes and Endocrinology,
Imperial College Healthcare NHS Trust,
London UK

Foreword by

David C Klonoff MD FACP FRCP(Edin) Fellow AIMBE
Medical Director, Diabetes Research Institute,
Mills-Peninsula Health Services,
San Mateo, California, USA

ELSEVIER

Edinburgh   London   New York   Oxford   Philadelphia   St Louis   Sydney   Toronto   2016

ELSEVIER

ISBN   9780702061240

British Library Cataloguing in Publication Data
A catalogue record for this book is available from the British Library

Library of Congress Cataloging in Publication Data
A catalog record for this book is available from the Library of Congress

Notices
Knowledge and best practice in this field are constantly changing. As new research and experience broaden our understanding, changes in research methods, professional practices, or medical treatment may become necessary. Practitioners and researchers must always rely on their own experience and knowledge in evaluating and using any information, methods, compounds, or experiments described herein. In using such information or methods they should be mindful of their own safety and the safety of others, including parties for whom they have a professional responsibility. With respect to any drug or pharmaceutical products identified, readers are advised to check the most current information provided (i) on procedures featured or (ii) by the manufacturer of each product to be administered, to verify the recommended dose or formula, the method and duration of administration, and contraindications. It is the responsibility of practitioners, relying on their own experience and knowledge of their patients, to make diagnoses, to determine dosages and the best treatment for each individual patient, and to take all appropriate safety precautions. To the fullest extent of the law, neither the publisher nor the authors, contributors, or editors, assume any liability for any injury and/or damage to persons or property as a matter of products liability, negligence or otherwise, or from any use or operation of any methods, products, instructions, or ideas contained in the material herein.

Content Strategist: Jeremy Bowes
Content Development Specialist: Helen Leng
Project Manager: Andrew Riley
Designer: Christian Bilbow
Illustration Manager: Amy Naylor
Illustrator: Graphic World Inc.

Printed in China
Last digit is the print number: 9 8 7 6 5 4 3 2 1

Contents

Contents

About the Authors

Dr Sufyan Hussain is specialising in diabetes with academic and teaching roles at Imperial College. He has strong clinical interests in type 1 diabetes. He is a type 1 diabetic himself with over 20 years' personal experience of using diabetes technology. His research has identified a key brain mechanism regulating glucose.

Dr Nick Oliver is a consultant diabetologist and clinical academic based at Imperial College London. He is an internationally recognised diabetes technology clinical researcher and leads a multidisciplinary clinical diabetes technology research group working with chemical, control and electronic engineers to develop future solutions for diabetes.

Foreword

Insulin pumps and continuous glucose monitors are two powerful tools and their use is increasing. They have been shown to improve blood glucose and haemoglobin A1c levels and to decrease low glucose levels at the same time. To use them properly it is necessary to understand diabetes physiology and the engineering that went into these products. This book makes it simple to understand how to use these two tools to improve diabetic glucose control. It fills an important need.

Written by two experienced diabetes physicians from Imperial College in London, a world class medical centre known for its advanced research in and excellent treatment of diabetes, Sufyan Hussain is an expert in finding treatments for diabetes that avoid low blood glucose levels and Nick Oliver is an expert in working with technology to develop a bio-inspired artificial pancreas that will someday control blood glucose levels without a need for testing glucose levels.

Reading *Insulin Pumps and Continuous Glucose Monitoring Made Easy* with its clear explanations, figures, tables, and case examples will help practitioners and patients get the most out of these important technologies.

David C. Klonoff

Preface

Technologies that support everyday living for people with diabetes are becoming more widely used. Continuous glucose monitors and insulin pumps are increasingly recommended to enable people to optimize glucose management. This book introduces these technologies to both general and specialist readers at any stage of their careers, providing a complete guide to insulin pump therapy and cases to illustrate the interpretation of continuous glucose monitoring.

The journey from multiple daily insulin injections to insulin pump therapy is covered in detail in the first section of the book, followed by the use of advanced pump features to ensure people using the technology get maximum value from it.

Chapter 1 introduces the reader to insulin pumps, indications, advantages and disadvantages of using this form of insulin therapy. It discusses the different types of pumps currently available. Chapter 2 discusses the details of initiating pump therapy with worked examples of how to calculate important settings. It details a frequently overlooked topic on selecting cannula, tubing length, inserting and wearing pumps. This chapter concludes with a detailed list of frequently asked questions and practical methods for troubleshooting.

Chapter 3 covers practical aspects of using pumps for daily activities such as eating and exercise. It covers the essential dosing method called carbohydrate counting and presents more advanced information on the effect of fat, protein, alcohol, coffee, fibre, and glycaemic index of a meal on blood glucose and using pump therapy in these settings. The chapter details the management of exercise with particular reference to hypoglycaemia avoidance during and following activity. Chapter 4, the final chapter in this section, presents practical advice on following up and managing special situations in insulin pump therapy. This includes optimizing pump settings, troubleshooting, downloading data from pumps, and managing difficult situations such as hospitalization, travel, sick days, pregnancy and stress. It also provides useful tips for structuring clinical services and pathways for pump therapy.

In the second section the sometimes tangled knots of continuous glucose monitoring are untangled with a guide to interpretation, examples of common traces, and chapters on real-time monitoring and sensor-augmented insulin pump therapy.

Chapter 5 is an introduction to the use of CGM devices. It explains how CGM works and covers different types of CGM. The chapter goes on to discuss clinical indications for using a CGM. It concludes with a practical discussion of how to insert a CGM into the body. Chapter 6 explains the steps that must be taken to obtain the most accurate and useful CGM results. These steps include proper calibration, setting and using threshold alarms and predictive alerts, and understanding trend arrows. Chapter 7 explains how to interpret CGM results using a six-part step-by-step approach, which is applied on an example CGM dataset and used to determine recommended actions.

In the remainder of the book (chapters 8-12), the step-by-step approach is used in a series of illustrated cases on different common topics in diabetes. These cases detail a clinical history, CGM data, interpretation of the data and recommended action plan to help guide the reader on interpreting CGM using the approach in Chapter 7. Cases increase in complexity with Chapter 8 covering basic common scenarios (non-diabetic, good and sub-optimal glucose control). Chapter 9 details frequent problems occurring at night such as low glucose levels (nocturnal hypoglycaemia) and rising glucose levels in the early morning hours (the dawn phenomenon). Chapter 10 covers use of CGM to manage glucose levels during four states of abnormal food intake: frequent snacking, alcohol intake, fasting and Ramadan. Chapter 11 includes the use of CGM for managing such glucose perturbing activities as exercise and shift work. Chapter 12 presents management of special situations using CGM. These include: high glycaemic variability, impaired hypoglycaemic awareness, pregnancy, bariatric surgery, and gastroparesis.

The final chapter, 13, covers sensor-augmented pump therapy, which combines the practices of measuring real-time CGM, reviewing CGM tracings, and reading insulin pump downloads. The chapter explains how most of these systems require input for insulin dosing by the patient but, in some new advanced systems, the pump will shut off insulin delivery in response to hypoglycaemia or impending hypoglycaemia. Two illustrated cases are presented.

This is the first book of its kind – designed to fill a significant gap in diabetes education and training. It combines theory with practical experience and illustrated examples. We hope that it is a useful companion to the increasing adoption of diabetes technology.

SH, NO

Acknowledgements

We would like to acknowledge the Imperial College Healthcare NHS Trust Diabetes Technology team and Dr Amir Sam for his support and contribution.

We are also extremely grateful to the helpful advice and comments provided by a number of colleagues, both professional and people with diabetes, whilst preparing this book.

We would like the thank the Elsevier publication team for its project management and administrative support that made this book possible.

Dedication

Nick – To A, B and E.
Sufyan – To A, I, M and Y.

Abbreviations

CGM	Continous glucose monitoring
CHO	Ingested carbohydrate
CSII	Constant subcutaneous insulin infusion
G	Pre-meal capillary blood glucose
GT	Target glucose
HBA1c	Glycated haemoglobin A1c
ICR	Insulin to carbohydrate ratio
IOB	Insulin on board
ISF	Insulin sensitivity factor
MAD%	Mean absolute difference as a percentage
MDI	Multiple daily injections
RT	Real-time
SD	Standard deviation
TBR	Temporary basal rate
TDD	Total daily dose of insulin
TDDi	Total daily dose of insulin on injections
TDDp	Total daily dose of insulin on insulin pump

An introduction to insulin pumps

1

Diabetes is characterized by a high blood glucose concentration and results from an absolute or relative deficiency of the hormone insulin. In type 1 diabetes, an absolute deficiency of insulin occurs due to autoimmune destruction of the beta cells of the Islets of Langerhans in the pancreas, which produce insulin. People with type 1 diabetes require insulin treatment that may be delivered by a regimen of multiple daily injections (MDI) or insulin pump therapy (also known as 'continuous subcutaneous insulin infusion' or CSII).

WHAT IS AN INSULIN PUMP?

An insulin pump delivers a pre-programmed amount of insulin at precise times. Insulin is held in a reservoir and is infused via an infusion set consisting of a flexible plastic tube (tubing) inserted into the subcutaneous tissue via a cannula (Fig. 1.1).

The pump delivers insulin in tiny amounts (microboluses), every few minutes over 24 h/day, hence the term continuous subcutaneous insulin infusion (CSII).

Soluble or rapid-acting insulin analogues are used. Insulin pumps deliver this insulin in two ways:
1. In a pre-programmed background amount
   – called a 'basal rate'.
2. In response to food eaten or high blood glucose concentrations immediately or over a specified period of time – called a 'bolus'.

WHY USE A PUMP?

Multiple daily injection regimens to treat type 1 diabetes require long-acting insulin of 1–2 injections per day (basal), and rapid-acting insulin injections before every meal or as a correction dose for high glucose (bolus). Understanding the differences between injections and pumps is important when considering why and when pumps should be used instead of injections.

HOW ARE PUMPS DIFFERENT FROM INJECTIONS?

Pumps have the ability to deliver tiny amounts of insulin over a planned time period. They can deliver small,

1

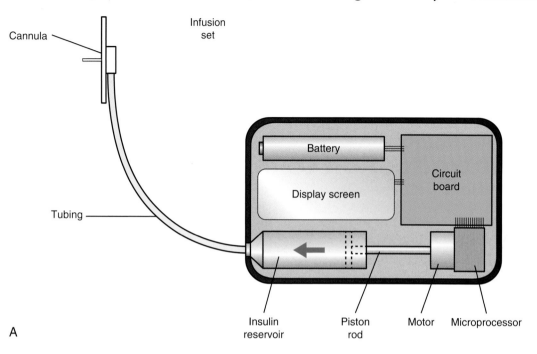

Cannula

Infusion set

Tubing

Battery

Circuit board

Display screen

Insulin reservoir

Piston rod

Motor

Microprocessor

A

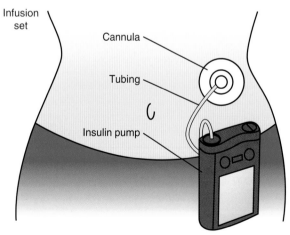

Infusion set

Cannula

Tubing

Insulin pump

B

2

Figure 1.1 Components of insulin pumps. (A,B) Computerized syringe or pump and infusion set consisting of tubing and cannula.

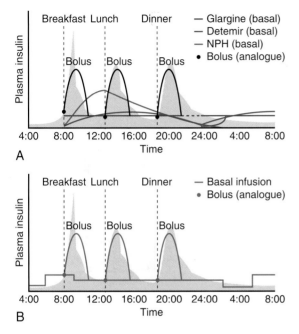

Figure 1.2 Basal insulin delivery for (A) basal-bolus injections and (B) insulin pumps compared. Shaded parts represent typical variable basal and different meal insulin requirements. Different basal profiles used in basal-bolus or MDI regiments are shown in (A). Unlike MDI regimens, insulin pumps (B) allow insulin delivery to be closely and conveniently matched to insulin requirements in people with diabetes.

pre-programmed doses of insulin without the need to insert a needle every time. This means that the insulin action (or pharmacokinetics) can be closely and conveniently matched to a person's insulin requirements. Variations in basal insulin requirements over a 24-h period are common (Fig. 1.2).

People often have reduced insulin requirement overnight, with increasing requirement on waking. The insulin pump basal infusion rate can be programmed to deliver insulin that fits that pattern in an individualized way. Similarly, basal rates can be reduced or discontinued with a pump at times of activity when insulin requirements are much lower. In contrast with MDI regimens, where rapid acting insulin can only be delivered once at the start of the meal, insulin pumps allow for mealtime boluses to be delivered over a prolonged period of time, enabling the insulin action to match the carbohydrate absorption with low glycaemic index foods.

Pumps can also deliver very small volumes of insulin with finer control over changes in insulin delivery. Insulin pen devices and syringes can typically deliver insulin in increments of 0.5–1 units, whereas pump increments are as low as 0.01–0.05 units. This is particularly useful for insulin-sensitive and very young people with diabetes.

The advantages and disadvantages of pumps over MDI are summarized in Table 1.1.

LIMITATIONS OF PUMPS (TO DATE)

While closed-loop insulin delivery systems are in development (sometimes called an 'artificial pancreas'), insulin pumps do not measure glucose concentrations and automatically adjust insulin delivery. Even sensor-augmented pumps (see Ch. 13) require blood glucose testing and manual adjustment of the pump to match insulin delivery to requirements.

Pumps cannot alter insulin action time ('on' and 'off' time) or pharmacokinetics. They do not deliver insulin directly into the bloodstream and are dependent on the time taken for rapid-acting insulin to be absorbed from subcutaneous tissue (typically 15–20 min). They are also dependent on the amount of time taken for a previously delivered dose of insulin to be used up. This means that even if a pump stops delivering insulin, insulin action may continue for some time. Even for rapid-acting analogue insulin, this is around 4 h, longer in certain situations, and varies from individual to individual.

Table 1.1 Summary of main advantages and disadvantages of pumps over multiple daily injections (MDI)

Advantages of pumps over MDI	Disadvantages of pumps over MDI
Fewer needle injections	**Constant attachment to pump**
No need to inject every time insulin delivery is required.	Must be worn all the time, including when asleep. Constant visibility and reminder of diabetes, which can affect perceived body image.
Insulin delivery can be conveniently varied, allowing more flexibility	**No long-acting insulin depot**
Basal rates can be varied and programmed to match activity, shift work, changing requirements (e.g. pregnancy, hormonal changes, growth spurts, illness, travelling). Bolus can be delivered over a varied time, e.g. pizza, malabsorption and gastroparesis. Temporary suspension or reduction of insulin delivery (activity and hypoglycaemia). Allows pre-programming of insulin to deliver variable amounts of insulin without constant input (e.g. while asleep or working).	Risk of rapid diabetic ketoacidosis development if technical failure or interruption in pump insulin delivery. Pumps can only be disconnected for short periods (e.g. swimming).
	Complicated set up – infusion set changes
	Set up for set changes is more complicated as compared to injections. Infusion sets and cannulas need to be changed every 2–3 days.
Small insulin doses	**Infusion set problems**
Deliver tiny doses (0.05–0.1 units) vs 0.5–1 unit in a syringe (useful for insulin-sensitive and young people).	Improper priming, air bubbles, tubing breaks and cannula kinks or slippages can interrupt delivery of insulin.
Overcome variations in insulin absorption	**Infusion site problems**
Long-acting insulin can be absorbed differently in different people. Delivering programmed basal rates tailored to individual needs overcomes this problem.	Uncommon but risk of skin infections.
Fewer snacks	**Increased education and training**
Tailored insulin delivery and reductions during hypoglycaemia and activity reduce the need for snacking.	Requires a higher level of education, understanding and motivation for the best use of the pump and to avoid problems.
Improved patient experience and satisfaction	**Increased healthcare provider training**
Improved self-management. Technology can motivate and improve engagement.	Healthcare providers need to have adequate knowledge and clinical systems in place to support pump therapy.
Better integration with technology	**Expense**
Newer pumps can link with other technology such as meters, continuous glucose monitors, bolus advisors, and diabetes information management systems.	Pump costs, as well as running costs (infusion sets, cannulas, batteries, accessories), are significantly more expensive than standard injections.

WHAT IS THE EVIDENCE FOR USING INSULIN PUMPS?

Meta-analyses of randomized controlled trials comparing insulin pumps with MDI in people with type 1 diabetes have shown the following advantages:

- Improved glycaemic control (HbA$_{1c}$) – the benefit in glycaemic control is more dramatic for a higher baseline HbA$_{1c}$
- Reduced frequency and severity of hypoglycaemia
- Reduced 24-h insulin requirements
- Reduced glycaemic variability, which may be associated with oxidative stress and endothelial dysfunction
- Improved quality of life and patient preference – more flexible lifestyle, improved energy, efficiency and confidence at work.

Better glycaemic control with reduced hypoglycaemia (allowing stricter control targets) is likely to reduce long-term diabetes complications.

Is there evidence for its use in other groups?

Insulin pump therapy is safe and may be a valuable treatment for people with insulin-treated type 2 diabetes, and preliminary data suggest that HbA$_{1c}$ improves with pump therapy. Current guidelines (which also incorporate cost–benefit estimates) do not advocate the routine use of pumps in type 2 diabetes.

There is anecdotal evidence suggesting benefits of insulin pump therapy for cystic fibrosis-related diabetes and pancreatic diabetes (pancreatitis and pancreatic surgery-related diabetes).

WHAT ARE THE BARRIERS TO PUMP THERAPY?

Although the evidence supporting pump therapy in type 1 diabetes is clear, there are some barriers to its widespread adoption:

1. *Cost of pump therapy*: The cost of pumps, consumables, accessories, replacements, set-up and training makes pumps more expensive than injections.
2. *User selection*: Pump therapy should be offered to those who will clinically benefit from it and who can make use of it. Offering pumps to people where it may not be used appropriately or where it may cause harm must be avoided (Ch. 2).
3. *Ensuring pump therapy is initiated and supported by a trained specialist diabetes team as part of a service*: Insulin pump therapy should be supported by a trained multidisciplinary pump team specializing in pump therapy (including a doctor, diabetes specialist nurse, dietician and access to a psychologist), who can provide structured education, with advice on diet, lifestyle and exercise suitable for type 1 diabetes.

WHICH PUMP SHOULD BE USED?

Insulin pumps vary in their size, interface, colour, complexity, simplicity and features. However, their unifying feature is the ability to program and deliver small doses of insulin over a planned time. Some additional features are now available (see Box 1.1).

WHAT ARE TETHERED PUMPS AND PATCH PUMPS?

There are two main sub-categories of insulin pumps: tethered and patch pumps (Table 1.2).

HOW TO CHOOSE BETWEEN TETHERED AND PATCH PUMPS

The main differences between patch pumps and tethered pumps are summarized in Table 1.3.

Box 1.1 Standard features in more recent pump models

- Small size
- Multiple cannula types (to suit different body types)*
- Bolus calculators
- Options to store and use multiple basal profiles
- Different bolus duration and shape
- Ability to link with glucose meters

- Ability to communicate with continuous glucose sensors
- Ability to wirelessly download pump data to a diabetes information management system
- Colour screens
- Simplified user interface

*not for patch pumps.

Table 1.2 Tethered and patch pumps

Pump type	Description	Use
Tethered pump (Fig. 1.1)	A long fine tube to connect the pump to the cannula. The pump is then worn and may be visible.	This is the most commonly used pump option as historically this is how pumps were designed.
Patch pump (Fig. 1.3)	A very short tube and cannula, which is integrated into a micro-pump device that attaches directly to the user. The pump is controlled via a handheld device.	A more recent design. More discreet. Integrated standard cannula (no variation possible)

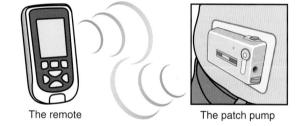

The remote   The patch pump

Figure 1.3 Patch pump. The handheld control device and patch micro-pump in place.

Table 1.3 Advantages and disadvantages of patch pumps over tethered pumps

Tubing	Minimal for patch pumps
Set changes	May be easier to perform with patch pumps as fewer steps involved.
Set issues	Lower risk of tube breakages or damage with patch pumps; however, it may be more difficult to visualize the cannula insertion point or monitor and remove air bubbles manually.
Size	Patch pumps may be more discrete.
Link to pump controls	Patch pumps are controlled via a handheld remote-control device. This wireless option is appealing to some and allows integration with capillary blood glucose meters. However, if the remote is lost or malfunctions, pump control may be very limited.
Continuous glucose sensor link	Currently, patch pumps do not have this feature but this may change in the future.
User preference	Patch pumps are popular due to their tubing-free design. Some users prefer a tethered pump because of other features, such as continuous glucose sensing and the ability to place the pump in different places without moving the cannula (e.g. on a belt, in a pocket and under the pillow).

FURTHER READING

Misso, M.L., Egberts, K.J., Page, M., et al., 2010. Continuous subcutaneous insulin infusion (CSII) versus multiple insulin injections for type 1 diabetes mellitus. Cochrane Database Syst. Rev. (1), CD005103.

Pickup, J.C., 2012. Insulin-pump therapy for type 1 diabetes mellitus. N. Engl. J. Med. 366 (17), 1616–1624.

Getting started with insulin pumps 2

GETTING THE FOUNDATIONS RIGHT

WHO BENEFITS FROM PUMP THERAPY?

Selecting the right user is key for successful pump therapy.

Clinical guidelines

Clinical guidelines provide useful criteria and indications for insulin pump therapy to guide healthcare professionals and people with type 1 diabetes. These guidelines take into account available evidence and cost–benefit analysis.

The UK National Institute for Health and Care Excellence (NICE) technology appraisal recommends pump therapy for people with type 1 diabetes who are:
- Unable to achieve target HbA_{1c} target of 8.5% or 69 mmol/mol with multiple daily injections (MDIs), including long-acting insulin analogues, despite a high level of care
- Experiencing disabling hypoglycaemia when attempting to reach target HbA_{1c} with MDIs
- Pregnant, if adequate glycaemic control is not obtained by multiple daily injections of insulin without significant disabling hypoglycaemia

- Children when MDIs are impractical or inappropriate.

Disabling hypoglycaemia is defined as: repeated and unpredictable hypoglycaemia, resulting in persistent anxiety about recurrence and an adverse effect on quality of life.

The Consensus statement by the American Association of Clinical Endocrinologists/American College of Endocrinology Insulin Pump Management Task Force provides the following criteria for insulin pump therapy in type 1 diabetes:
- HbA_{1c} >7.0% or 53 mmol/mol
- Increased blood glucose fluctuations before meals
- 'Dawn phenomenon' with fasting glucose >11.1 mmol/L or 200 mg/dL or significant glycaemic excursions.

User characteristics

Insulin pump therapy is a powerful adjunct to education, support and motivation in improving both glucose and quality of life outcomes in type 1 diabetes. To achieve optimal outcomes, prior to embarking on pump therapy potential users should:
- Regularly engage with health services and professionals

9

- Self-manage their diabetes as effectively as possible
- Use carbohydrate counting, making insulin dosing adjustments appropriately with food and to correct blood glucose
- Use an optimal multiple daily injection regimen with insulin analogues
- Be able to perform required pump adjustments
- Understand the risks of insulin pump therapy
- Perform regular self-monitoring of blood glucose (at least ≥4 per day).

As a long-term condition, diabetes may be associated with distress, depression or anxiety. Psychological support may be critical to enable pump therapy to improve outcomes. The multidisciplinary team should be involved in insulin pump initiation. In addition to clinical visits, structured education programmes and saline pump trials offer useful opportunities to evaluate suitability for pump treatment.

How should pumps be selected?

Different types of pumps are covered in Chapter 1. Local availability may limit pump selection. As a general rule, selection should take into account the points in Table 2.1.

PROGRAMMING THE PUMP

HOW TO START INSULIN PUMP THERAPY

Starting people on insulin pump therapy requires a working knowledge of how to convert injection insulin doses to pump settings.

Which insulin?

In most cases fast-acting insulin analogues are preferred given their quicker on and off times. Remember, even analogues take some time to start working and work for several hours (Table 2.2).

Table 2.1 Selecting the right pump

Individual preference and choice	Remember the person with diabetes will be using and wearing the pump continuously! Individual choice of pump may be important in getting the best results.
Healthcare professional experience	Healthcare professional experience with differing pumps may vary and expert support and education is important in supporting the long-term goals of pump therapy.
Technical and consumables support	Availability of technical support, a replacement pump service in case of faults and upgrades may be important considerations.
Additional features	Depending on user requirements, such as ability to link with a continuous glucose sensor (sensor-augmented pump therapy) or being waterproof.

Table 2.2 Pharmacokinetics of quick-acting insulins

	Onset	Peak	Duration
Analogue insulin (e.g. aspart, lispro and glulisine)	15 min	50–90 min	2–5 h
Soluble human insulin	30 min	2–4 h	Up to 8 h

The durations are indicative; there is significant inter- and intraindividual variation that will alter the action of insulin.

What basal rate should be used initially?

The total daily dose of insulin administered with pump therapy is generally slightly lower than with an MDI regimen. There are several ways to calculate the initial basal rates on insulin pump therapy, including using the basal insulin dose of multiple injections, the total daily dose of multiple injections or using circadian infusion rates derived from physiology data.

The total daily dose method is frequently used and illustrated here:

Step one – estimate the average amount needed per hour

1. Calculate the total daily dose of insulin on injections (TDDi).
2. Reduce the TDDi by 20% to give the total daily dose on insulin pump therapy (TDDp).
3. Divide this by 2 to give the total daily basal insulin dose on pumps.
4. Divide this by 24 h to give the amount needed per hour.

Worked example 2.1: Calculating the initial basal rate

A 28-year-old woman with type 1 diabetes is reviewed in the Diabetes clinic. Her HbA$_{1c}$ is 75 mmol/mol (9%) despite multiple daily injections and a high level of care. Her current insulin regimen consists of:

- Insulin aspart: 5–7 units with breakfast, 3–5 units with lunch and 5–7 units with the evening meal
- Insulin glargine: 14 units before bed

Calculated initial basal rate:

1. Calculate mean total daily dose on MDIs (TDDi):

$$6+4+6+14=30$$

2. Reduce the total daily dose (TDDi) by 20% to give the total daily dose of pumps (TDDp):

$$20\% \text{ of TDDi}: 0.20 \times 30 = 6$$

$$\text{TDDp}: 30 - 6 = 24$$

3. Divide the TDDp by 2 to give the total amount of basal insulin: 24/2 = 12
4. Divide by 24 to give the hourly rate: 12/24: 0.50

Basal rate 0.50 units/h (round down if needed).

Step two – refine to the individual's needs

The above method does not take into account variations in basal requirements. There is good evidence to suggest that as a result of general circadian rhythm, meal and activity levels, basal needs in most people will change (see Fig. 2.1 and Table 2.3).

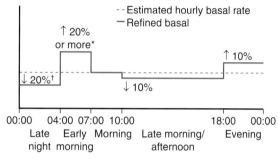

* Higher needed if marked dawn phenomenon. Lower if risk of night time hypoglycaemia
† Lower if risk of night time hypoglycaemia

Figure 2.1 Adjustments in basal rates to take into account, in usual circadian rhythm, activity and meal patterns.

Table 2.3 Changing basal needs

Time period	Change	Adjustment to basal
Late night (00:00–04:00)	Reduced on average	Reduce calculated amount by 20%.
Early morning (04:00–07:00)	Increased due to dawn phenomenon and breakfast	Increase calculated amount by 20% (higher if marked dawn phenomenon).
Morning (07:00–10:00)	No change	No change.
Late-morning and early afternoon (10:00–18:00)	Possible slight reduction due to increased activity with effects from breakfast and lunch bolus	Reduce calculated amount by 10%.
Evening (18:00–00:00)	Increased with dinner and sedentary behaviour	Increase calculated amount by 10%.

Worked example 2.2: Refining the calculated basal rate

The person with diabetes in worked example 2.1 has a calculated basal rate of 0.50 units/h. If she is at risk of overnight hypoglycaemia and dawn phenomenon, the calculated basal can be modified as follows:

Table 2.4 The calculated basal rate

Time	Calculation	Basal settings (per hour)
00:00–04:00	$0.5 - (0.5 \times 0.2) = 0.4$	0.4 units
04:00–07:00	$0.5 + (0.5 \times 0.2) = 0.6$	0.6 units
07:00–10:00	0.5	0.5 units
10:00–18:00	$0.5 - (0.5 \times 0.1) = 0.45$	0.45 units
18:00–00:00	$0.5 + (0.5 \times 0.2) = 0.55$	0.55 units

The variation will deviate depending on the individual schedule (such as shift and activity patterns), and further adjustments can be made.

Further considerations

In addition, calculated insulin requirements from injection dosages may be higher if the starting HbA_{1c} is high and if there is low risk of hypoglycaemia. With experience, the reduction in TDDi can be lowered to account for this.

Table 2.5 Basal features on pumps

Basal profiles	Use different profiles for days with different levels of activities or insulin requirements. For example, profiles may be set for weekdays and weekends, to manage hormonal changes, such as premenstrually and during intercurrent illness.
Temporary basal rate	Use to increase or decrease the basal rate for short periods (0–8 h). This is useful to adapt dynamically to circumstances. A temporary reduction in basal infusion may be used during exercise or following alcohol consumption and a temporary increase in basal rate may be used during, e.g. illness or stress.

A higher reduction in TDDi may be needed if there is a high risk of hypoglycaemia, loss of hypoglycaemia awareness or a history of severe hypoglycaemia.

Some software packages will calculate initial circadian basal infusion rates. These are based on physiological data and fine tuning is likely to be needed.

Basal features on pumps

Pumps also have the ability to set different basal profiles and temporary basal rates (Table 2.5).

Table 2.6 Ways to estimate insulin:carbohydrate ratios

Rule	Who	Calculation	Formula
'500 rule'	Most adults	500 divided by the calculated pump total daily insulin dose	500/total daily dose on insulin pump therapy (TDDp) = amount of carbohydrates covered by 1 unit of insulin
'300 rule'	Pre-school children	300 divided by the calculated pump total daily insulin dose	300/TDDp = amount of carbohydrates covered by 1 unit of insulin

How much to bolus with meals?

Most insulin pumps have insulin bolus dose calculators integrated into them, which will calculate an insulin dose to match ingested food and to correct hyperglycaemia. These require several personalized parameters, which are:

- Insulin:carbohydrate ratio (ICR)
- Insulin sensitivity factor (ISF)
- A glucose target (GT).

The bolus dose is calculated using the equation:

$$B = \frac{CHO}{ICR} + \frac{G - G^T}{ISF} - IOB,$$

where B is the insulin bolus dose, CHO is the ingested carbohydrate, G is the pre-meal capillary blood glucose, and IOB is insulin on board. IOB is derived by the pump depending on the amount of insulin it has delivered over the preceding few hours (see p. 14).

Insulin:carbohydrate ratio (ICR)

This reflects the amount of insulin needed for the amount of carbohydrates consumed. Ways to estimate this are shown in Table 2.6.

Worked example 2.3: Calculating ICR

Using the doses in Worked example 2.1, where the pump total daily dose (TDDp) = 24 units (p. 11).

Table 2.7 Calculating insulin:carbohydrate ratio

'500 rule' (Adults)	'300 rule' (young children)
'500 rule': 500/24 = 20.83 Round to 20 g carbohydrate ICR is 1:20 This means that 1 unit of insulin is required for every 20 g of carbohydrate consumed	'300 rule': 300/24 = 12.5 ICR is 1:12.5 or 13 g. This means that 1 unit of insulin is required for every 12.5 or 13 g of carbohydrate consumed

The ICR is programmed into the pump. Some pumps can program different ICRs for different times. Many people need more insulin for a given amount of carbohydrate at breakfast. Again, fine tuning is needed.

Insulin sensitivity factor (ISF)

The insulin sensitivity factor describes the predicted drop in blood glucose after 1 unit of insulin is given. This can be estimated using the '100 rule' if using mmol/L or the '1800 rule' if using mg/dL for glucose measurements.

- '100 rule': 100 divided by total daily insulin dose on insulin pump
- '1800 rule': 1800 divided by total daily insulin dose on insulin pump

---

Worked example 2.4: Calculating ISF

Using Worked example 2.1, where total daily insulin dose on pump (TDDp) is 24 units.

Table 2.8 Calculating insulin sensitivity factor

Rule: (TDDp = total daily dose on pump)	'100' rule for mmol/L 100/TDDp	'1800' rule for mg/dL 1800/TDDp
Using Worked example 2.1 (where TDDp = 24 units), ISF =	100/24 = 4	1800/24 = 75
1 unit of insulin will reduce the blood glucose by:	4 mmol/L	75 mg/dL

This too may need fine tuning if hypo- or hyperglycaemia is recurrent after meals or after glucose corrections.

Active insulin time and Insulin on-board (IOB)

Active insulin time reflects the amount of time a given dose of insulin continues to work after it has been delivered. It is set to ensure the bolus calculator can estimate the 'on board' or active insulin. Most typically, it is set at 4 h. It can be increased or decreased to address recurrent hypo- or hyperglycaemia after meals or after correction doses. Shorter IOB times means the pump will only include the effect of more recent insulin administered and there is a risk that the insulin on board effect will be underestimated. This can result in insulin 'stacking', where a bolus acts in addition to a previous bolus, which will result in lower than desired glucose levels and a higher risk of hypoglycaemia. This is why it is usually appropriate to set this feature for 4 h or longer. If the IOB is set for a duration over 4 h, then the effect of insulin on board may be overestimated, resulting in smaller boluses and higher than desired glucose concentrations.

The active insulin time is particularly increased in people with impaired kidney function, as up to 80% of insulin is cleared by the kidneys. It also changes with the amount of insulin dose, weight and if human or animal insulins are used.

Blood glucose targets

These will vary from individual to individual. The pump uses inputted targets to work out the amount of insulin needed when using its bolus advisor. Different targets can be set for different times to ensure optimal personalized glucose control.

DIFFERENT BOLUS OPTIONS

Pumps have the ability to deliver three main bolus types: normal or standard bolus; square-wave or extended bolus; dual-wave or multi-wave bolus (also known as combo bolus) (see Fig. 2.2 and Table 2.9).

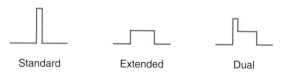

| Standard | Extended | Dual |

Figure 2.2 Different bolus types.

Table 2.9 Different bolus types

Bolus type	Explanation	Use
Normal or standard bolus	Bolus insulin is delivered immediately.	Normal meal or correction (similar to bolus insulin injection).
Square-wave or extended bolus	Bolus insulin is delivered over an extended, defined period of time.	Low glycaemic index foods, such as porridge. High fat meals, which slow the absorption of carbohydrate (such as pizza or curry).
Dual-wave or multi-wave bolus	A combination of normal bolus and square-wave/extended bolus.	Large carbohydrate meals or separate courses. Delays in digestion such as from gastroparesis.

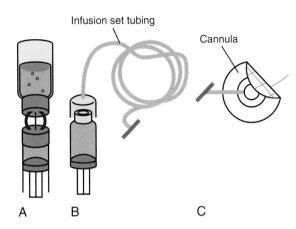

Figure 2.3 Infusion set and reservoir connects insulin, pump and user.

How to use dual- or multi-wave boluses?

1. Use the bolus calculator or manually calculate the total bolus required.
2. Divide the bolus into the percentage to be given immediately (this is usually around 30–50%). The remainder will be given over a longer period of time.
3. Determine the time period for the extended bolus (this is usually 2–4 h but may be longer).
4. The extended or square bolus can be stopped at any time.
5. It is important to remember that the temporary basal feature cannot be used while dual- or multi-wave bolus is operating.

   An example of using a dual- or multi-wave bolus with food is shown in Worked example 3.2 (p. 26).

WEARING A PUMP

Pump therapy requires the user to be connected to a device delivering insulin almost all of the time. Setting up infusion sets and wearing the pump correctly is critical for good outcomes with pump therapy.

WHAT IS AN INFUSION SET AND RESERVOIR?

Pumps have a tank of insulin called a 'reservoir'. This is connected to the user via tubing that attaches to a cannula inserted subcutaneously. The reservoir, tubing and cannula are collectively called 'the infusion set' (Fig. 2.3).

WHICH CANNULA?

Cannulas are available in different materials, may be inserted manually or with an inserter and are angled at 45° or 90°.

Table 2.10 Advantages and disadvantages of soft and steel cannulas

Type	Description	Advantage	Disadvantage
Soft cannula	Made of Teflon®, a flexible plastic material. Introduced subcutaneously via a metal needle, which is removed, leaving the plastic cannula in the skin	May be more comfortable. Recommended for people with nickel allergies.	May kink or be bent under the skin, which can slow insulin delivery.
Metal or steel cannula	Harder	Kink or bend less. Easier to insert. Useful in situations where reliability is desired due to lower risk of cannulas slipping out or bending (e.g. pregnancy).	May be less comfortable. Change every 48 hour (rather than 72 hours)

Soft or steel cannula?

Advantages and disadvantages of soft and steel cannulas are summarized in Table 2.10.

Angled or 90° soft cannulas?

The point of skin entry of the cannula needle can be angulated or perpendicular (90°) to the skin (Fig. 2.4).

The advantages and disadvantages of angled or 90° cannula insertion are summarized in Table 2.11.

What cannula length and gauge?

Cannulas for different types of sets come in different lengths. The 90° cannulas are 6–12 mm in length, while angled cannulas are up to 17 mm long.

Generally, longer length cannulas have less risk of slippage but an increased risk of being inserted into the muscle. Longer cannulas are recommended in people with a higher body mass index (BMI); frequent issues with cannula slippage; lipohypertrophy or higher insulin requirements (≥25 unit boluses or ≥2.5 units/h basal).

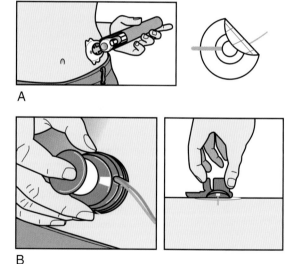

A

B

Figure 2.4 Angled cannula and insertion device.

Table 2.11 Advantages and disadvantages of angled or 90° cannula insertion

Type	Description	Advantage	Disadvantage
Angled (20–45°)	Longer cannula inserted at an angle	May be better for leaner pump users. Angle can be fine tuned by user. Window at the insertion point in the adhesive dressing (so user can see whether the catheter is inserted in the skin). May be less prone to kinking and falling out.	Can be harder to insert in difficult to reach areas or if visual or manual dexterity problems.
90°	Shorter cannula inserted perpendicular to the skin	Useful if insertion is desired in difficult to reach areas (arm, buttock or hip). Often done with the aid of an insertion device. Less visibility of the needle – good if user has fear of needles.	Risk of inserting into muscle in lean people. Less visibility of needle to confirm successful insertion.

The gauge of the needle refers to its thickness (with smaller gauges being thicker). Usual sizes are between 25 gauge (thicker) and 27 gauge (finer). Larger gauges may be more suited to people with a higher BMI or where there may be a risk of kinking or bending.

Which tubing length?

Tubing lengths are usually between 24 and 42 inches. The user's height (taller adults may need longer tubing), where they choose to wear the pump and placement of the pumps while sleeping, changing clothes, exercising or using the washroom, all influence which length to use.

Which tube disconnection mechanism?

There will be times when pump users need to disconnect themselves from the tubing and pump, while leaving the cannula inserted (e.g. showering, exercise, swimming, times of intimacy). To facilitate this, there are various disconnection mechanisms. The two main types are 'twist and lift off' and 'sideways pull disconnection' mechanisms. The former is easier to disconnect, but harder to reconnect in difficult to access areas. The latter has a 'click' to indicate appropriate reconnection but requires more dexterity.

In addition to the above, a secondary disconnection point in the tubing further away from the point of insertion is sometimes available and is useful for difficult to access insertion points.

Which reservoir?

There may be options for different reservoir sizes. The standard 1.5–2 mL size is applicable to most people, as it can hold sufficient insulin to last 72 h and allows the reservoir to be changed at the same time as the rest of the infusion set. The larger 3 mL size is useful for people with a higher insulin requirement, to avoid more frequent reservoir changes.

HOW DO WE GET THE PUMP CONNECTED WITH THE INSULIN?

Draw the insulin into the reservoir

This is similar to drawing up a syringe with a vial. Air bubbles must be expelled. Room temperature insulin makes drawing up without air bubbles easier.

Prime the tubing

The tubing needs to be connected to the reservoir. Pumps have a mechanism to prime the tubing with insulin and ensure the pump's piston head (that pushes insulin out of the reservoir) is firmly pressed against the reservoir plunger. During this process, air bubbles must be expelled.

Insert the cannula

Figure 2.5 shows the potential places to insert the cannula, which are similar to the injection sites.

Site rotation is critical and either an M or W method or clock method should be used (Fig. 2.6). The new site should be at least 2.5 cm away from the previous site, avoiding the waistband or 2.5 cm from the umbilicus.

Tips

Adhesive sprays, barrier dressings or anaesthetic creams can be used to improve the security of the cannula, prevent allergy and reduce discomfort.

For men, shaving the desired site helps to ensure proper contact with the cannula adhesive and reduces risk of slippage.

Bleeding into the cannula lumen suggests that the cannula may be positioned in or near a blood vessel and may need to be removed as insulin absorption may be different.

After insertion, there may be slight stinging but if this persists beyond 30 min and especially with movement, as the cannula may be in a muscle. Removal and reinsertion of the cannula is suggested.

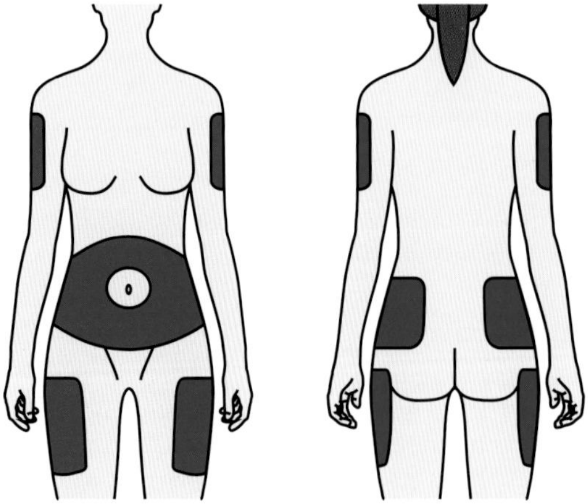

Figure 2.5 Sites for cannula insertion with pumps.

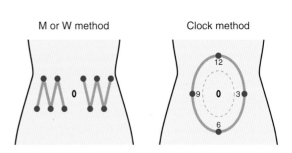

Figure 2.6 M or W and clock methods for rotation of cannula insertion sites.

Connect the pump and prime the cannula

Attach the pump tubing to the cannula. At this point, the cannula has a small amount of dead space. Most pumps have an automated feature to fill this; alternatively a manual bolus may be needed. The exact amount varies with cannula type (0–1 unit) and should be checked.

Now that the pump is connected, convenient options for wearing the pump continuously need to be considered. Pumps come with a belt clip or pouch with a clip that allows them to be worn on trousers. A small hole cut into a trouser pocket to feed the tubing through can be considered. Bra straps or thigh pouches can be used to hold the pump and a wide range of accessories is available, including garters, pouches and harnesses, to fit different pumps. Some devices have remote-control options to control the pump if worn in a difficult to access place.

What about patch pumps?

Priming and inserting the pump is still applicable to patch pumps, with the main exception being that there is no or only very short tubing. The priming and insertion processes are often more automated. When wearing a patch pump, it is important to consider that it will be in place for up to 72 h, so a site compatible with the next few days' activities should be selected. No disconnection is usually needed.

PROBLEMS

Problems with setting up and wearing the pump are one of the leading causes of unexplained high blood glucose on pumps. Frequent issues are listed in Table 2.12.

Other common issues include pumps running out of insulin or batteries running down.

Good pump practice is needed and the following should be encouraged:
- Check the infusion site and tubing at least daily (and see Table 2.12)
- Change the site every 2–3 days to reduce risk of infection and degradation of insulin in hot temperatures
- Clean the insertion site to allow good adhesion and shave if needed
- Rotate your site regularly
- Always have close access to a spare reservoir, infusion sets, insulin and batteries at all times (even for day trips)
- If in doubt, re-draw new insulin into a new reservoir and perform a set change (attach new tubing and insert a new cannula).

FREQUENTLY ASKED QUESTIONS

Pump users will naturally face a number of situations, which may not have obvious answers. The most frequently asked questions are shown in Table 2.13.

Table 2.12 Frequent problems with wearing insulin pumps that can lead to high sugars

Problem	Possible remedies
Cannula slipping out or dislodged	Ensure skin is adequately prepared and cleaned (including shaving if needed). Different cannula length or type may be needed if a recurrent problem. Additional adhesive may be needed (sprays or dressing), especially if excessive sweating. Ensure tugs on tubing are not a cause of this, in which case different length tubing could be helpful.
Tube breakage	Ensure tubing length is not too long.
Air bubbles	Visibly inspect tubing and reservoir. Expel air bubbles if needed. Ensure insulin and infusion set are at room temperature when filling and priming.
Site infection	Watch out for tenderness, redness, warmth, inflammation (swelling) at the site of insertion. Remove and replace infusion set. If fever, discharge, drainage, lump (abscess) or persisting features, seek medical attention.
Skin reaction to adhesive	Some people with sensitive skin may get irritation, redness, rash and itching with the cannula adhesive. Using a different adhesive type (if available), or a dressing under the adhesive (to prevent skin contact) with a larger more suitable dressing over the site to secure the cannula, may help.
Lumps at insertion site	Possible reasons could be incorrectly sited cannula, large insulin doses, reaction to insulin or site infection (if other features as above). Ensure sites regularly rotated. Avoid lumpy sites (prolonged rest periods). Consider longer or shorter cannula.
High glucose before set change	May reflect prolonged set or reservoir use. Ensure infusion set and new insulin is drawn up more regularly, especially in hot environments.
Tube or cannula blockages	Rare but can happen with insulin crystals forming. Most pumps will alarm if they are unable to deliver insulin (failed delivery alarm). Reservoir with fresh insulin and a set change usually corrects this.
Bolus or suspend due to accidental button presses	Rare, as most pumps feature alarms for insulin suspension and have safety features to prevent this (button lock-out and multiple steps needed).

Table 2.13 Frequently asked questions about wearing insulin pumps

Question	Answer
What should I do when I am sleeping?	Pumps can be kept clipped or strapped. Some people prefer having them off straps or clips (e.g. under the pillow). Tubing needs to be long enough to allow this and can get tangled if turning around but this should not impair delivery of insulin.
Will the tube, cannula or pump compress if I roll over during sleep?	Pumps and tubing are extremely durable and do not compress with normal daily use. Cannulas do not compress either, but sleeping on them can be uncomfortable.
What should I do if I shower?	Disconnecting the pump from the infusion set and re-inserting after the shower is the best option. Same applies for sauna and steam rooms. (Remember hot temperatures can accelerate insulin absorption.)
What should I do if swimming or on the beach?	See activity section (p. 28 and Table 3.2) for swimming. For prolonged periods over 4 h, periodic bolus doses may be used or revert to multiple dose insulin injection regimen.
What should I do during exercise/sports?	See activity section (p. 28 and Table 3.2).
What should I do during periods of intimacy?	Disconnect pump from the infusion set. Do not remain disconnected for periods over 2 h. You can keep the pump in 'suspend' mode so it alarms in case you fall asleep and forget to reconnect.
Do I need any special precautions during MRI scans?	Pumps or any electrical device should not be exposed to strong electromagnetic fields, as it may damage them. Therefore, they must be disconnected and left outside the scanner room. If a metal cannula is used, it must be removed prior to the scan.
Do I need any precautions when going through X-rays or airport security?	Most modern pumps are safe to wear when going through security X-rays. However, it is best advised to check this with the device manufacturer. (If in doubt, remove.) For strong energy fields, such as medical X-rays or CT scans, it is advisable to disconnect from the insulin pump. Steel cannulas can be left in place.

FURTHER READING

AACE/ACE, 2014. Consensus statement by the American Association of Clinical Endocrinologists/American College of Endocrinology insulin pump management task force. Endocr. Pract. 20 (5), 463–489.

NICE. Continuous subcutaneous insulin infusion for the treatment of diabetes mellitus. NICE technology appraisal guidance [TA151]. 2008 (modified 2014). Online. Available: http://www.nice.org.uk/guidance/ta151.

NICE. Diabetes in pregnancy: management of diabetes and its complications from preconception to the postnatal period. NICE guidelines [NG3] 2015. Online. Available: https://www.nice.org.uk/guidance/ng3.

Eating and activity with pumps

EATING WITH PUMPS

Food needs to be matched with appropriate amounts of insulin for optimal diabetes control. Carbohydrates have the biggest impact on blood glucose. Carbohydrate counting provides an accurate and flexible approach that is particularly suited to fast acting insulin analogues and pumps.

CARBOHYDRATE COUNTING – THE BASICS

There are three main types of carbohydrate: starch, simple sugars and fibre. Starch and sugars are converted to glucose on digestion. The body does not break down fibre. In its simplistic form, carbohydrate counting assumes that starch and sugar will cause a rise in glucose (Fig. 3.1). This needs to be matched with insulin according to the insulin:carbohydrate ratio (ICR) (p. 13). There are also other variables,

which are discussed later. When starting to learn pump therapy, focussing on basic carbohydrate counting (accurately measuring portions, determining carbohydrate content and using this with pumps) is advised.

HOW DO WE CARBOHYDRATE COUNT TO DETERMINE INSULIN DOSE?

1. *Determine the carbohydrate content of food*: Use the nutrition label, reference list and serving size determination to calculate total carbohydrate.
2. *Determine the insulin needed for food*: This is the total carbohydrate eaten multiplied by the insulin needed per gram of carbohydrate.
3. *Determine the insulin needed for correction of glucose*: This is glucose reading subtracted from target or ideal glucose. Divide this by the insulin

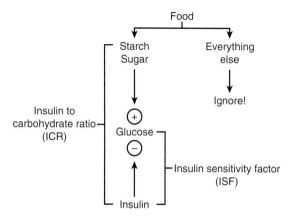

Food

Starch
Sugar

Everything
else

Ignore!

Insulin to
carbohydrate ratio
(ICR)

⊕
Glucose
⊖

Insulin sensitivity factor
(ISF)

Insulin

Figure 3.1 Basic carbohydrate counting. Starch and sugar are broken down to glucose. Only these are counted in grams when calculating insulin using the insulin to carbohydrate ratio (ICR). If the glucose levels are high, a correction dose of insulin can be given at the same time, using the insulin sensitivity factor (ISF).

sensitivity factor (ISF). Remember, if the glucose level is lower than the target, a reduction in bolus may be needed.

WHEN TO GIVE INSULIN IN RELATION TO MEALS?

Rapid acting insulin analogues should be given 15 min before eating (p. 10, Table 2.2). This can be difficult when timing of meals or amount eaten is less predictable (e.g., eating out, children, hyperemesis in pregnancy). Unlike MDI, pumps allow a portion of the bolus to be conveniently given 15 minutes before meals, with the remainder taken just before or after the meal is eaten as a compromise in less predictable situations.

Worked example 3.1

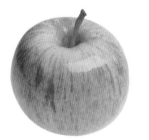 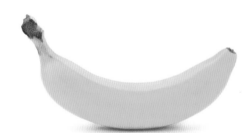

With a blood glucose of 11 mmol/L (target 6 mmol/L), one small apple and one medium banana are eaten (Fig. 3.2). The ICR is 1 unit: 10 g and ISF is 1 unit:2.5 mmol/L. What is the insulin dose required?

- Carbohydrate content of food = 15 (apple) + 20 (banana) = 35

- Insulin needed for food = total carbohydrate eaten × ICR = 35 × 0.1 = 3.5 units
- Insulin needed for correction of high glucose = (current glucose–target glucose)/ISF = (11 − 6)/2.5 = 2 units
- Total insulin = bolus for food + corrective dose = 3.5 + 2 = 5.5 units

WHAT IS NEEDED FOR CARBOHYDRATE COUNTING TO WORK?

1. *Correct basal, ICR and ISF*: these need to be worked out and correct if carbohydrate counting is to work.
2. *Nutritional label*: standardization of nutrition labels in the North America and Western Europe has made it much easier to keep track of carbohydrate content in foods which can be read on the label. Calculation of the carbohydrate in the serving size may need to be made, as carbohydrate amounts are often expressed as 100 g of food rather than serving size.
3. *Carbohydrate reference lists*: easily available from structured learning programmes, online or nutrition reference or facts books and smartphone apps. A variety of popular foods are included. There may be some list to list variation. Not required if nutrition label is available.
4. *Serving size*: in some cases, this is easy to work out, for example with bread slices, pizza slices or fruit. In others it requires objective accurate measurements with food measures. This is usually needed for foods, such as rice, pasta, cereals, mashed potato, which are difficult to quantify with the eye alone and are high in carbohydrate content. Initially, food scales and with practice, measuring cups and spoons can be used. The carbohydrate values of cooked and raw foods can vary and lists will distinguish this. Remember precise measurements mean precise insulin doses. Small errors can affect blood glucose.
5. *Arithmetic skills or a calculator*: carbohydrate counting does require good simple arithmetic skills to work out carbohydrate content and insulin doses.
6. *Use your pump and insulin correctly*: for simple carbohydrate counting, remember that even with rapid acting analogue insulin the optimal time to bolus is around 15 min before food. Taking it correctly will prevent glucose spikes. (Other options for delivering insulin are discussed later.)
7. *Accurate record-keeping and frequent blood glucose monitoring*: essential to understand whether the approach is working or needs refinement. Few attempts may be needed to understand if it is working correctly.
8. *Patience, persistence, practice and perseverance*: necessary to get carbohydrate counting to work. It is daunting and may not work the first few times but does get easier.
9. *Refresh skills*: good behaviours need reinforcement. Refresher courses and revision of skills are helpful in maintaining this.

WHAT ABOUT OTHER VARIABLES?

A number of other important dietary and non-dietary variables that can affect blood glucose are not taken into consideration. It is difficult to factor in every variable given the complexity of human physiology.

The focus of this chapter is on understanding how to use pumps with food. Other variables that have a strong effect on insulin action, such as activity and exercise, illness, menstrual periods, fasting, are discussed in detail separately.

DOES FAT IN FOOD CHANGE BLOOD GLUCOSE?

Large, high fat meals, such as a pizza or curry, can increase the time for digestion, resulting in longer absorption times for carbohydrates. High fat meals can also result in the body being more resistant to insulin after several hours. Therefore, after a high fat meal, glucose tends to rise later. An immediate bolus could result in an initial fall in glucose followed by delayed hyperglycaemia. Ways to overcome this are to use dual- or multi-wave bolus options, typically taking anywhere between 30% and 70% of the bolus amount immediately and the remaining over 2–4 h.

Worked example 3.2

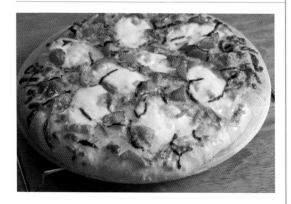

With a blood glucose of 6.0 mmol/L (target 6 mmol/L), half a 12 inch deep pan pizza or 4 pizza slices are eaten (120 g carbs) (Fig. 3.3). The ICR is 1 unit:10 g and ISF is 1 unit:2.5 mmol/L. What is the insulin dose required?

- Carbohydrate content of food = 120 g
- Insulin needed for food = total carbs eaten × ICR = 120 × 0.1 = 12 units
- Insulin needed for correction of high glucose = (current glucose-target glucose)/ISF = 0
- Total insulin = bolus for food + corrective dose = 12 units
- Large quantity, high fat food therefore delayed absorption expected. Using dual/multi-wave option:
  - 6 units now (normal bolus)
  - 6 units over 4 h (extended or square wave bolus).

WHAT ABOUT GI (GLYCAEMIC INDEX)?

Glycaemic index (GI) determines how quickly a carbohydrate acts to increase blood glucose. It is scored on a scale of 100, with pure glucose being 100. Slowly absorbed foods have a low GI rating, typically <55. Foods that are more quickly absorbed have a high GI rating, typically >75. The GI index helps with working out timing of insulin boluses and understanding post-meal hyperglycaemia, but does not influence the amount of carbohydrate. It therefore complements carbohydrate counting and if used in conjunction with this, can achieve better control.

For example, insulin should be taken more than 15 min before eating high GI sugary foods to avoid a sharp glucose rise immediately post-meal. Low GI foods with high fat and fibre results in glucose being released slowly and a dual- or multi-wave bolus may be needed.

What are low and high GI foods?

There are comprehensive lists for glycaemic index. A number of variables affect it (including cooking, processing, physical form or coatings, acidity, fat or fibre content), and individual variation in speed of digestion with high pre-meal glucose and large meals also slowing digestion. Therefore, learning lists is not of great value. What is useful, however, is recognition of GI index as a variable when assessing post-meal glucose values, adjusting insulin times, type of bolus and amount accordingly.

Fibre

Fibre is not digested and therefore not turned to glucose. For carbohydrate counting, subtract fibre from the total carbohydrate content if >5 g in a serving is coming from fibre.

Protein

Protein can result in glucose rises several hours after a meal, as amino acids which make up protein can be metabolized to form new glucose molecules, particularly during periods of fasting. Protein may have a protective effect, reducing the frequency of post-meal hypoglycaemia. Carbohydrate-free protein snacks and meals may need a small insulin bolus but validated ways to calculate the insulin to protein ratio are not available.

Alcohol

Alcohol can have a large impact on glucose levels. It can reduce glucose release from the liver resulting in hypoglycaemia, often hours after alcohol. It is recommended that a snack containing carbohydrate should be taken without a bolus to slow alcohol absorption and prevent hypoglycaemia. Alternatively, a temporary basal rate may be used after alcohol to reduce the insulin effect, particularly in the liver. At the same time, high sugar content in alcoholic beverages may cause a rise in glucose while drinking.

Learning and refining from experience is the best way to determine how to manage glucose, which will respond differently to different beverage type and the quantity drunk. It is advisable to use no or smaller bolus initially (reduce ICR by half), monitor frequently, set alarms to wake-up to test and advise others of the risk of going low and what to do if this happens.

Coffee

In addition to the carbohydrate content of milky caffeine beverages, coffee can cause a degree of insulin resistance so that a larger amount of insulin may be needed as a temporary basal rate or bolus with food. This varies from person to person.

Tips

Everyone responds differently. It is important to practise good record-keeping and regular reviews to determine how the body responds to different dietary variables. Food diaries with record of bolus doses, timing and basal rates may be helpful when embarking on pump therapy and determining how to use it effectively to manage glucose with food. Smartphones with time-stamped pictures of food eaten provide another way of doing this with pump data downloads (see p. 34).

ACTIVITY WITH PUMPS

Exercise and activity are very important for people with diabetes. However, activity requires insulin delivery adjustments to avoid hypo- and hyperglycaemic excursions. These depend on the level and nature of exercise and can be easier to manage with pumps.

WHAT HAPPENS TO GLUCOSE DURING EXERCISE?

During exercise, the glucose consumption increases to meet the increased energy demands from muscle. This consumption can be very dramatic for intense exercise, especially in the first 10 min. There is also an increase in cutaneous blood flow that accelerates insulin absorption. Hence, during exercise, there is a significant risk of hypoglycaemia. After exercise, the muscle insulin sensitivity is increased, making it more responsive to insulin and glucose consumption is higher as it replenishes its glycogen stores. Therefore, there is also an increased risk of hypoglycaemia following exercise and insulin requirements are reduced for up to 24 h.

The extent of the above depends on the level, duration of exercise and also fitness of the person. Furthermore, very intense, or anaerobic exercise can cause a paradoxical rise in blood glucose mediated by adrenaline and counter-regulatory hormones to insulin during and after exercise. Hyperglycaemia during exercise adversely effects muscle performance and there is an increased risk of dehydration and ketosis with hyperglycaemia.

A few general rules are worth following:
1. Start slowly and build up. As tolerance improves, and the body's strength and glycogen stores increase, you may find that the body responds differently.
2. Keep glucose with you at all times.
3. Avoid exercise if ketones are present.
4. Stay well hydrated.
5. Check glucose before exercise (2 h prior and immediately before), 30–60 min into exercise and after exercise.

Planning ahead – temporary basal, carbohydrate loading and reduced bolus

As more glucose will be utilized during exercise, insulin needs to be reduced and additional carbohydrate may be needed to maintain glucose before and after exercise (Table 3.1).

These approaches may be used in combination and personal preference, timing of exercise and blood glucose levels before exercise will dictate which is used.

WHAT TO DO AFTER EXERCISE

The increased risk of hypoglycaemia after exercise can last for 24 h. This may be especially problematic overnight.

Following significant exercise, the following can be tried:
1. Reduce temporary basal rate by 20–50% for 2–4 h.
2. For the next 24 h, a separate basal insulin programme with a smaller reduction (of around 20%) in basal insulin is advised. The biggest period of reduction is in the overnight basal rate.
3. The ICR following exercise may be reduced to reduce insulin boluses. Either 15–20 g extra carbs

Table 3.1 Approaches to prevent hypoglycaemia during exercise		
Approach	**Explanation**	**Description**
Approach 1 – reduce temporary basal rate	Basal insulin levels can be reduced prior to, during, and after a period of exercise.	Reduce basal insulin by up to 50%, start 60–120 min before exercise and maintain the reduction during the exercise.
Approach 2 – carbohydrate loading	Altering basal rates before exercise may not always be possible. Fast acting carbohydrate immediately prior to intense short activity may be helpful. For longer, moderate intensity, a slow releasing solid snack may be better.	Take 15–20 g extra carbohydrates without an insulin bolus before exercise.
Approach 3 – reduced bolus	Take a reduced bolus with meals prior to exercise.	If eating a meal within 2 h prior to exercise, reduce the bolus dose by 25–75%.

or a 20% reduction in bolus insulin may be needed with the main meal following exercise.

4. Check capillary blood glucose regularly after exercise.

Table 3.2 summarizes common problems during exercise, the reasons for them and ways to correct them.

Table 3.2 Common problems and solutions during exercise

Problem	Explanation	Solutions
Immediate hypoglycaemia during or just after exercise	Due to increased glucose consumption during exercise. Symptoms of hypoglycaemia such as sweating may be masked due to exercise.	Reduce basal settings further prior to exercise and ensure reduction is at least 90 min before exercise. Take extra carbohydrate before or during depending on when the hypoglycaemia occurs. Test during the exercise period or use continuous glucose sensing to get a better understanding of glucose change and action that is needed.
Delayed overnight hypoglycaemia	Due to recovery and replenishment of glycogen with increased insulin sensitivity.	Reduce overnight basal further, consider setting an alarm and testing during the night or using continuous monitoring. If the hypoglycaemia is in the first half of the night, consider reducing insulin taken with dinner or use bed-time snacks.
Post-exercise hyperglycaemia	Intense and anaerobic activity may trigger stress responses. This coupled with reduced basal rates could lead to hyperglycaemia after exercise. In some cases, this may be very marked. It can lead to dehydration and ketosis, which can impair the recovery period after exercise.	Ensure well-hydrated during exercise, test immediately after and take a correction insulin bolus, which may be higher than usual due to the presence of counter-regulatory hormones to insulin. To prevent in future, minimize basal reductions during exercise, test during exercise and give a 50% corrective bolus if high.
Contact sports	With some contact sports there is a risk that the cannula or pump may be dislodged.	Remove pump for periods up to an hour. After an hour, test capillary blood glucose, take required carbohydrate and insulin and continue exercise.
Swimming	Some pumps can be worn when swimming and will deliver a basal throughout swimming.	Pumps can be removed and cannulas can be left attached. It is recommended that it is removed in non-chlorinated environments to avoid risk of infection. The cap for the cannula and a dressing can be worn if left attached to the body. If the pump is removed for over an hour, test capillary blood glucose, take required carbohydrate and insulin and continue swimming.

Mastering the insulin pump 4

WHAT AND WHEN TO RECORD

Pump users should be encouraged to record and review their bolus, basal, carbohydrate, blood sugar and activity in log sheets. Alternatively, these data can be automatically logged in pumps, or even smartphone apps, and downloaded (p. 34). This can be essential for optimal pump therapy, allowing review of patterns through which trends and problems can be determined and fine tuned.

HOW TO CALCULATE BASAL AND BOLUS CORRECTLY

Which is to blame – basal or the bolus?

Identifying the contribution of basal and bolus insulin to recurrent hyper- and hypoglycaemia can be difficult. Basal rate testing may identify issues with the basal rates and continuous glucose monitoring can suggest mismatch between insulin and food. Changes to insulin should be made sequentially as multiple changes can make it difficult to know which has been successful

and the impact of changes should be reviewed over several days.

Generally, consider the basal amount or timing needs adjustments for:
- Blood glucose variations (low or high) during the night or before breakfast
- Low or high glucose if a meal is delayed or skipped.
Consider the bolus (including the ICR and ISF) for:
- High or low glucose within 4 h of a bolus or meal
- Hypoglycaemia following a correction insulin bolus.

BASAL RATE TESTING

Blood glucose levels are affected by a number of variables including:
- Basal insulin
- Food (carbohydrate) intake
- Bolus insulin – mealtime and correction boluses
- Activity
- Factors, such as stress or illness.
Basal rate testing is a process that examines the insulin pump basal rate, while trying to eliminate or

minimize the influence of other factors. The simplest way to do this is to divide the day in several time windows where people are following a normal routine with no strenuous activity preceding or during the period of testing and not taking any carbohydrates (ideally fasting for the entire period). This allows normal state basal requirements to be determined. An example of a protocol is given below. Basal rate testing can be performed and repeated as often as required. Timings can be varied and test periods can be focussed on problem times.

Basal rate testing protocol

General guidelines:
1. Ensure the person is well with no hypoglycaemia in the last 12 h.
2. No carbohydrate (ideally no food or drink other than water) should be consumed during the period of testing.
3. Ensure the person is following a normal routine, with no strenuous activity in the preceding 24 h, no increased activity during the period of testing and not experiencing an increase in stress.
4. Use current basal rates.
5. Stop testing if blood glucose falls below 4 mmol/L or 70 mg/dL, and treat for hypoglycaemia.
6. Stop if blood glucose increases above 14 mmol/L or 250 mg/dL, and take corrective bolus.
7. Record blood glucose, basal rate, carbohydrate content of food before or after and any other variables.
   Do basal testing on one of the following windows (repeat for remaining windows on different days):
   Overnight basal testing (21:00–07:00):
1. Basal testing window between 21:00 and 07:00.
2. Evening meal before 19:00, after which no further food (ensure evening meal is easy to carbohydrate count to avoid errors in carbohydrate counting impacting testing window).
3. Test blood glucose at 21:00, 00:00, 03:00 and 07:00.
4. Usual breakfast and bolus at 07:00.
   Morning basal testing (07:00–12:00):
1. Basal testing window between 07:00 and 12:00.
2. Proceed only if fasting glucose in target and omit breakfast.
3. Test blood glucose at 07:00, 09:00 and 12:00.
4. Usual lunch and bolus at 12:00.
   Afternoon basal testing (12:00–18:00):
1. Basal testing window between 12:00 and 18:00.
2. Proceed only if pre-lunch glucose in target and omit breakfast.
3. Test blood glucose at 12:00, 14:00, 16:00 and 18:00.
4. Usual evening meal and bolus at 12:00.
   Evening basal testing (18:00–22:00):
1. Basal testing window between 18:00 and 22:00.
2. Proceed only if pre-dinner glucose in target and omit dinner.
3. Test blood glucose at 18:00, 20:00 and 22:00.
4. Evening meal and bolus at 22:00.
   Evaluating and adjusting insulin during basal testing:
- Adjust basal rate by 0.025–0.1 unit/h (10–20% increase or decrease).
- Adjust if blood glucose varies, increases or decreases by 1.5 mmol/L or 25 mg/dL during a 4 h period.
- Adjust 1–2 h before blood glucose change.

Assessing basal rates using continuous glucose monitoring

Basal rates may be assessed using continuous glucose monitoring to record glucose values during times of fasting or low carbohydrate intake. This can be assessed using retrospective continuous glucose monitoring or real-time monitoring. In the event of hypoglycaemic or hyperglycaemic symptoms, the pump users should test their capillary blood glucose and take appropriate action.

To ensure appropriate interpretation of continuous glucose monitoring, an event diary should be completed, including meals, capillary blood glucose and insulin doses, including basal rates, mealtime bolus and correction bolus. During the period of monitoring, normal basal rates should be used.

HOW TO ENSURE BOLUS DOSES ARE CORRECT

If the basal rate is tested and corrected, looking for problems in the bolus becomes more straightforward. When analysing pump data, glucose excursions 2–4 h after a bolus may be addressed if other factors are ruled out. The meals at the end of the basal tests provide a useful picture of the ICR if a 2- and 4-h blood glucose test is undertaken.

Possible problems with glucose after bolus insulin are summarized in Table 4.1.

Table 4.1 Reasons for problems with glucose after bolus insulin

Bolus calculation	Check log book/food diaries for errors. Check arithmetic. Bolus calculator use minimizes errors.
ICR	Assess using simple/easy to count meals. Remember ICR can vary during different times of the day.
Carbohydrate counting	Check in clinic with visual aids/prompts. Smartphone pictures or food diaries can help.
ISF	Look for impact of correction doses on glucose when other variables are not changing.
Other factors	Other variables, as discussed earlier.

TROUBLESHOOTING HYPOGLYCAEMIA

Reasons for hypoglycaemia
See Table 4.2.

Treating hypoglycaemia
People with diabetes and their carers should be advised as follows:
1. Keep pump running.
2. Test before treating.
3. Take 15 g fast-acting carbohydrate.

Table 4.2 Reasons for hypoglycaemia

Reasons	Solutions
Inappropriate targets for blood glucose	Adjust targets on bolus calculator.
Infrequent blood glucose monitoring	Test at least 4–6 times per day.
Overestimating carbohydrates	Check and refresh carbohydrate counting. Check insulin to carbohydrate ratios.
Too large bolus with food or different bolus type needed	Use reduced and/or multi-wave or extended bolus.
Slow digestion	Use multi-wave or extended bolus.
Basal rate too high	Basal rates: test regularly.
Over correction/frequent corrections (insulin stacking)	Avoid repeat bolus or use calculator.
Alcohol	Eat with alcohol. Use reduced temporary basal.
Stress	Use temporary basal.
Exercise	Use reduced temporary basal, snack if needed.

4. Re-check blood glucose in 10–15 min.
5. If not corrected, repeat fast-acting carbohydrate and consider temporary basal reduction 10–20% (especially if recurrent or severe hypoglycaemia).

Training to enable prevention and self-management of hypoglycaemia should be provided to everyone with type 1 diabetes.

TROUBLESHOOTING HYPERGLYCAEMIA

Reasons for hyperglycaemia

See Table 4.3.

Treating hyperglycaemia

Treatment guidance can be given to treat hyperglycaemia as shown in Figure 4.1. If there is no improvement or worsening ketosis and high glucose, emergency medical assistance must be sought immediately.

Table 4.3 Reasons for hyperglycaemia

Reasons	Solutions
Infection, illness, stress	Sick-day rules (see pp. 36–37)
Basal rate too low or reduced activity	Increase basal insulin.
Steroids	See pages 36–37
Pump problems	See page 20, Table 2.12
Insulin omission or insufficient insulin	Bolus to be taken 15–20 min before meals; adjust ICR if needed.
Over treatment of hypoglycaemia	Check hypoglycaemia treatment.
Pump failure	Contact pump company, revert to injections and await replacement pump.

DOWNLOADING PUMPS

Most pumps allow data to be uploaded, analysed and displayed in easy to understand and interpret formats. The use of bolus calculators where food and blood glucose data may be entered, linked glucose meters and use of other pump features allows visualization of basal, bolus, food, carbohydrate counting, behavioural patterns, as well as other very useful data during clinic visits or remotely. There are also a number of smartphone apps that allow data entry and logging.

These data can support optimal outcomes from insulin pump therapy. People with type 1 diabetes may also upload their data and obtain periodic advice from the multidisciplinary team remotely via telephone or e-mail.

WHAT IS NEEDED FOR PUMP DOWNLOADS?

Below are some suggestions for making the best use of information from pump downloads:
1. *Download before or during the clinic visit prior to consultation.* Downloading pumps in the clinic usually requires having relevant software installed and cables/transmitters available. It also takes time and therefore having a system to ensure this can be done is important. Pump users may be able to upload their own data before visits or bring printouts with them but it helps to have facilities at the clinic to do this.
2. *Reviewing data.* This takes practice and familiarity with the way the data are presented. In general, the below approach can be considered.

HOW TO ANALYSE DATA

Basic information

1. Insulin information:
   a. Pump programs – basal profiles, ICR and ISF can be viewed.

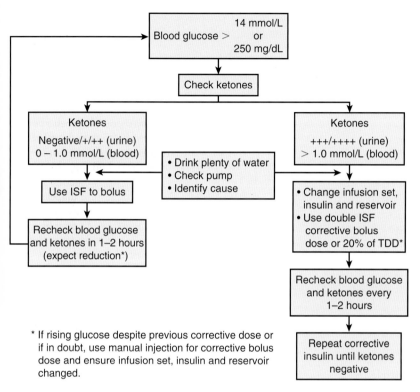

Figure 4.1 Treatment of hyperglycaemia with insulin pumps.
- Can take ~ 4 hours to normalise
- Be aware of insulin stacking and risk of hypoglycaemia with multiple doses to correct
- If there is no improvement or worsening ketosis and high glucose seek emergency medical help immediately

b. Basal:bolus ratio – although it is difficult to make generalizations, a 50:50 or 40:60 ratio is typical. The basal may be lower if the person is very active. Large deviations from this ratio may prompt consideration of whether the correct basal or bolus doses are being used.

c. Amount of insulin used per day.

2. Glucose data:

a. Average tests: at least 4–6 times/day is expected with pumps.

b. Percentage high and low: can give a glimpse of how much time is being spent outside the desired range and in hypoglycaemia. This will be overrepresented if people test more when they 'feel' high or low.

3. Average carbohydrate intake: usually around 200 g/day but varies.

4. Set changes: every 2–3 days.

Trends

This relies on looking at the pooled average glucose data and spotting obvious trends. Although we are used to doing this with glucose diaries, looking at a large amount of data graphically provides a much more powerful way of doing this. It also allows visualization of glucose patterns against basal, bolus and meal patterns to make adjustments to therapy. When looking to pick up trends, it is useful to break up the day into the following windows:

- Overnight period
- Breakfast to lunch
- Lunch to dinner
- Dinner to bed-time.

Exceptions

These are extreme highs and lows, which affect people most. They are often reflective of issues concerning:

- Correction of hyperglycaemia (overcorrection or stacking leading to hypoglycaemia)
- Errors in carbohydrate counting
- Missed or miscalculated boluses
- Set change problems (if delayed leading to highs)
- Unanticipated activity or stresses.
  Simple trends to look out for:
- Overnight glucose control
- Hypoglycaemia (time/preceding activity/bolus)
- Glucose control after hypoglycaemia (reflects correct correction)
- Hyperglycaemia
- Glucose control after hyperglycaemia (reflects correct correction)
- Pre-meal glucose control
- Glucose control after meal
- Glucose control after exercise.

UNPLANNED SITUATIONS

People with diabetes will run into situations that they cannot always plan for. One of the essential aspects of pump therapy is to know how to handle unanticipated tricky situations. The main feature to manage all these

and more situations is careful monitoring, logging, reviewing and adjusting.

ILLNESS AND 'SICK DAYS'

Illnesses will increase counter-regulatory stress hormone secretion. This will increase insulin requirements with an associated increase in risk of hyperglycaemia (which can worsen dehydration) and ketosis. If vomiting or where there is poor oral intake, there is a risk of hypoglycaemia. The following general tips may be of use:

1. Always take insulin – never stop or suspend your insulin pump. Extra insulin may be needed for moderate or severe illnesses (Table 4.4).
2. Stay well hydrated (aim for at least 100 mL/h).
3. Check blood glucose every 1–4 h (more frequently in severe illnesses).
4. Check blood or urine ketones if vomiting, poor intake or if blood sugar is above 14 mmol/L (250 mg/dL) and treat as shown in Figure 4.1.
5. Keep a log of glucose, insulin, ketones, fluids, vomiting and temperature if possible.
6. Eat if possible – try to eat simple, digestible foods if unable to tolerate complex meals.
7. Some treatments may also impact on glucose (e.g. steroids, which are used in acute exacerbations of asthma or chronic obstructive pulmonary disease).
8. Let others know that you are unwell.
9. Seek urgent medical attention if vomit is continuous, if you are unable to eat and drink or if you have continued high glucose or ketones.
10. If in doubt, ask for help.

STEROIDS

Corticosteroids, such as prednisolone, dexamethasone and hydrocortisone, are given for inflammatory and

Table 4.4 Sick-day rules with pumps

	Minor illness (common cold, cough)	Moderate/severe illness (pneumonia or diarrhoea and vomiting)
Blood glucose testing	4–6-hourly	1–2-hourly
Basal rate	No change needed unless prolonged illness or hyperglycaemia, in which case consider 10–20% basal increase.	May need 30–50% increase in basal rate (check glucose to determine trend, start temporary basal at 130% and increase if needed). If vomiting or poor oral intake and glucose dropping, may need to reduce basal by 30% – do not stop insulin.
Bolus	No change – correction dose as needed unless ketones (see below).	
Ketones	Blood 1.5–3.0 mmol/L (urine +/++). 10% total daily dose insulin bolus (may need to repeat 2-hourly if ketones or hyperglycaemia persists). Increase basal by 30%. Blood >3 mmol/L (urine +++/++++). 20% total daily dose insulin bolus (may need to repeat 2-hourly if ketones/hyperglycaemia persists). Increase basal by 50%.	
End points	If rising glucose despite previous corrective dose or if in doubt, use manual injection for corrective bolus dose and ensure infusion set, insulin and reservoir changed. If ongoing vomiting, unable to drink, unable to control glucose or ketones despite above – seek urgent medical help as an emergency.	

autoimmune conditions (e.g. asthma and inflammatory bowel disease) and may also be used in other settings. High doses of corticosteroids cause insulin resistance and will increase insulin requirements dramatically. Depending on which steroid is used, hyperglycaemia will occur at differing times of day. To cover for this:

- An increase in basal of 30–50% initially may be needed during times of maximal hyperglycaemia. Increases of up to 200–300% are not uncommon
- ICR may also go up; however, to keep things simple this may be left unchanged and corrective insulin can be taken if needed
- A close log (4–6 hourly) of blood glucose should be kept to work out individual requirements

- As steroids are reduced or stopped, insulin requirements can drop back very quickly and adjustments are needed.

STRESSFUL SITUATIONS

Stressful situations are much like sick days with stress responses, which are counter-regulatory to insulin action. There is significant interpersonal variation in how blood glucose reacts to the same stress, with direction, magnitude and duration of glucose change all differing between people with diabetes and scenario.

For short-duration stressors, a temporary basal increase can be used 2 h before the event, if it can be anticipated. Increases may be conservative (10–20%) to avoid hypoglycaemia, which can impair performance and additional small correction boluses can be used to address any remaining hyperglycaemia.

For long-duration stressors, a higher basal pattern over a period of weeks may be needed. Frequency of capillary blood glucose testing may increase to ensure hypo- and hyperglycaemia are avoided, as these may exacerbate stress and can affect performance. Insulin requirements can drop quite sharply after the stressful period is over and reduced basal patterns may be needed.

MENSTRUAL CYCLE

Women with type 1 diabetes may experience high glucose levels and increased insulin requirements during the premenstrual period, which may require a different basal profile or may be managed with temporary basal rates. When menstruation starts and progesterone concentrations fall steeply, insulin requirements may fall sharply and there may be a higher risk of hypoglycaemia. Most women may not notice a change in their glucose levels with oral contraceptive pills. However some women may report a slight increase in basal insulin requirements, particularly with older high-dose contraceptive pills or depot progesterone injections.

TRAVEL

Travelling with a pump is straightforward but requires planning.

Things to prepare before travelling – general advice:
- Ensure you have all your supplies – not just pump supplies and insulin but blood glucose and ketone monitoring, rapid acting glucose supplies, glucagon kit, back-up syringes and long-acting insulin

- Keep supplies in a bag that stays with you at all times (cabin baggage). Extra pump reservoirs, infusion sets and batteries can be kept in check-in luggage. If possible, give a smaller back-up supply to someone travelling with you in case luggage is misplaced
- For long-distance travel or travel in hot countries, keep insulin in an insulation bag, such as an evaporative cooling case
- Ensure you keep documentation from your doctor confirming you have type 1 diabetes and need to carry supplies with you and need to wear your pump at all times – this may be needed for airport security
- Know where to obtain medical help if needed and keep key contact numbers
- Locating and obtaining pump supplies can be a problem in some countries
- Medical travel insurance is advised and ensures it covers your diabetes and pump use
- If travelling in a group, make sure group members are aware that you have diabetes and what they may need to do in an emergency
- Keep any reminders you may need, such as your pump settings, sick-day rules, multiple dose injection doses.

Insulin adjustments when travelling

Making insulin adjustments for time changes can be challenging. The pump (and blood glucose meter) clocks can be adjusted to change the basal rates but it may take several days for circadian rhythms to re-establish to a new time zone. Therefore, variable basal rates to match circadian patterns may initially be timed incorrectly. The following general guidance can be given:
- Use a lower basal rate while travelling for the first 24 h (10–20% lower)
- Change the time on your pump to the new local time when you arrive at your destination

- Frequent capillary blood glucose testing may be required initially

You may need extra attention if:

- The time zone changes more than 3 h
- There is significant baseline variability in basal rates – such as for marked dawn phenomenon
- There is reduced hypoglycaemia awareness or a history of recurrent or severe hypoglycaemia.

One strategy to optimize adjustment to a new time zone is to make pump clock adjustments in stages – by 2–3 h/day – and use a lower basal setting with frequent self-monitoring.

When and how to come off pump therapy

People with type 1 diabetes may wish to stop pump therapy for short periods, such as to go on a beach holiday or due to a pump malfunction. A documented plan should be provided and reviewed regularly to enable this.

Changing to subcutaneous injections

To work out how much long-acting basal insulin is needed – the following approximation may be used:

- Calculate the total daily basal insulin on the pump program
- Increase this by 20% to determine the amount of long-acting insulin needed per day (a 30% increase may be needed, but a conservative 20% increase is advised at first)
- This can be given as one dose or two doses, depending on which insulin is being used and total insulin dose
- The pump should be discontinued 2 h after the first long-acting insulin injection is given. It is best to do this in the morning to minimize the risk of problems at night
- Bolus insulin and corrective doses should be taken as usual. If a bolus calculator is used, the one on

the pump can still be used or a calculator integrated into a capillary blood glucose meter can be used.

Resuming pump therapy

When resuming pump treatment, return to previous pump settings. The best time to restart this is just before the long-acting insulin has worn off (approximately 2 h prior to the next due dose of long-acting insulin). It is advisable not to do this just before bedtime as close monitoring is advisable after re-starting pump treatment.

SPECIAL SITUATIONS

CHILDREN

Insulin pumps can improve glucose control in childhood and have the potential to overcome many of the challenges of a multiple daily dose regimen with finer control of insulin doses, a reduced frequency of subcutaneous injection, greater personalization and the potential for caregivers to make changes to insulin administered without using needles. Management of insulin pump therapy in childhood requires additional education to carers, as well as to the child and this can be challenging.

School

Management of type 1 diabetes in school children requires clear communication between healthcare professionals, the child, carers and school staff, to ensure safe, effective diabetes management during school time. Insulin pump therapy can be self-managed by many children at a young age but, in case of pump failure, insulin should be kept at school in a fridge with needles and syringe or insulin pen, and school staff should be familiar with supporting hypoglycaemia treatment.

PUBERTY

Adolescence and young adulthood is a difficult time due to hormonal and body changes, psychological changes and environmental changes. This is a period when insulin requirements change in a manner that is difficult to predict and will require close supervision for adjustments to achieve stable control. Often insulin requirements increase during puberty, partly due to growth, but also as a result of increased insulin resistance mediated by an increase in the concentration of sex hormones.

PREGNANCY

Optimal glucose control during pregnancy minimizes the risk of large-for-gestational age babies and associated complications affecting both the mother and baby. However, achieving optimal glucose control can be challenging in the context of nausea and vomiting in early pregnancy and with dynamic increases in insulin requirement as the normal insulin resistance of pregnancy advances. Insulin pump therapy can support intensification of glucose during pregnancy, while avoiding distressing hypoglycaemia. The progression to pump therapy occurs ideally before pregnancy to avoid destabilizing glucose control while pregnant but pump therapy can be commenced during pregnancy if hypo- or hyperglycaemia are difficult to address with MDI regimens. Routine surveillance of infusion sites and set changes are advised given the high risk of accidental ketosis in pregnancy. As the abdomen stretches, other sites or a steel cannula can be considered to minimize the risk of cannula dislodgement.

Breast-feeding

Insulin requirements during breast-feeding fall significantly (by up to 25%), as available carbohydrate is used to provide lactose in milk. Managing this change in insulin requirement soon after delivering a baby can be particularly challenging, as it is superimposed on the reducing insulin requirements, which are associated with no longer being pregnant. Insulin pump therapy may enable rapid reductions in insulin requirements during this period and during breast-feeding. The use of temporary basal rates can reduce the risk of hypoglycaemia.

HOSPITALIZATION

Where possible, people with type 1 diabetes on insulin pump therapy should be empowered to continue to self-manage their diabetes during a hospital admission. Healthcare professionals should be aware and comfortable with this. Sick-day rules may be needed with higher basal rates and this can be supported by the multidisciplinary team.

If pump therapy is discontinued or removed, subcutaneous basal insulin or intravenous insulin infusion must be used.

Diabetic ketoacidosis treatment

Ketoacidosis should be managed according to local guidelines. It is important to ensure that pump failure or problems with insulin delivery via the pump were not the precipitant of ketoacidosis. If the insulin pump was disconnected, the pump can be restarted once the ketoacidosis has been treated (avoid starting this overnight). Intravenous insulin infusion should be continued for a further 1–2 h before stopping.

Outpatient procedures

No adjustments may be needed if basal rates are set up correctly. Blood glucose should be monitored closely as insulin requirements may go up (due to stress of the procedure) and sometimes fall (due to missed meals and if basal rates were not correct).

Surgery

For elective surgery, basal insulin via pump may be continued but careful consideration of management of the pump while under anaesthetic is required. A variable rate intravenous insulin infusion should be considered and factors in the operating theatre, such as diathermy and its impact on the pump, may influence this decision. For emergency surgery, it is likely to be safest to stop insulin pump therapy, store the pump safely and commence a variable rate intravenous insulin infusion.

Labour and delivery

If diabetes is stable, and the woman or her partner are able to manage the insulin pump, it may be continued through labour. If problems arise with glucose or the labour, the infusion set can be removed and a variable rate intravenous insulin infusion can be commenced. The insulin requirements will sharply decline after delivery due to a fall in pregnancy hormones and breast-feeding. There is an increased risk of hypoglycaemia and basal rates should be reduced to below pre-pregnancy settings with frequent glucose monitoring.

PATHWAYS FOR PUMP INITIATION AND MANAGEMENT

An insulin pump clinical service may include the following pathways:

PRE-PUMP

The education and support of people working towards insulin pump therapy is key to successful outcome. The pre-pump part of a pump service should include:

Structured education for insulin dose adjustment

To derive optimal glucose outcomes from pump therapy, people with type 1 diabetes must be able to carbohydrate count, manage activity and illness and should be able to alter insulin in response to their blood glucose trends.

This can be delivered via structured education programmes or by other means, such self-education, online resources, interactive training and peer support. Structured or supplementary education should be offered to anyone with diabetes prior to initiation with pump treatment. On rare occasions, initiation of insulin pump therapy may be clinically urgent and the requirement for education may be less important.

Pump trials

Saline pump trials may be a useful way of assessing an individual's suitability for insulin pump treatment, allowing the pump user to address, and potentially alleviate any concerns regarding wearing the pump. Saline trials may also act as an additional educational tool.

Managing expectations

Starting pump therapy can be a frustrating experience with potential for an initial period of worsening glucose control. It also involves an intensive period of learning and errors may occur. Whilst support in the initiation phase of pump treatment is key, it is extremely important to explore peoples' expectations prior to pump therapy. They must be realistic and achievable to avoid frustration and disengagement.

PUMP INITIATION

The following general considerations are useful to optimize pump initiation:

Saline trials

- Where indicated.

Initiation sessions

- This requires focussed training, usually by a specialist diabetes educator. The initial session can take 2–4 h and intensive follow-up may be needed
- Can be in groups or individual. The support of peers and a shared experience can be very positive
- If appropriate, carers and family should be involved
- Must be done in an appropriate setting. Education should be provided on:
  - Setting up the pump: setting changes, inserting cannulas, drawing up insulin, troubleshooting
  - Using the pump: bolus, basal, temporary basal, using bolus advisors, suspending pump, main functions and changing general settings
  - Managing carbohydrate counting and using bolus advisor
  - Managing hyperglycaemia with pumps and troubleshooting
  - Managing hypoglycaemia with pumps
  - Where and how to access help and support.
  Written information should be provided on the above.

Support for initiation

This can be intense and requires a lot of learning. The following methods may be of help:
- Contact details of diabetes specialist nurses, pump companies and other helpful contacts (e.g. buddy groups, online resources) should be provided
- A follow-up plan should be detailed to ensure correct usage, provide further education and for correcting any problems
- Ensure an appropriate support network is in place with time and space to adapt to pump therapy.

Specialist and increased monitoring at initiation

This may be needed for certain groups, such as:
- Pregnant women (close review needed)
- People with active diabetic retinopathy (review retinopathy within 3 months of initiation recommended)
- Reduced hypoglycaemia awareness, recurrent or severe hypoglycaemia.

Example of pump start protocol

Following a pump start:
- 1st day after pump start, check glucose 2-hourly and continue this overnight
- Correct blood glucose >14 mmol/L or >250 mg/dL with a correction bolus as advised
- Treat blood glucose <4 mmol/L or 70 mg/dL
- Daily telephone follow-up with diabetes/pump nurse for 1–2 weeks
- Within first 2 weeks, carry out basal rate testing for 24 h period and make appropriate adjustments
- Within 1 month, diabetes/pump nurse follow-up in clinic
- 1st review in pump clinic usually 3 months after starting pump therapy, then a minimum of twice annually if stable.

PUMP FOLLOW-UP AND SUPPORT

Clinic follow-ups

Ongoing advice and care from a specialist team is needed. This can be complemented with virtual clinics (telephone, video) or e-mail. There is no consensus on frequency of follow-up, which varies depending on clinical need. In addition to routine diabetes care, the follow-up in a pump clinic may additionally focus on:
- Reviewing the clinical and pump data (blood glucose, test results, insulin requirements and pump settings)

- Providing further education
- Setting goals of pump therapy
- Ensuring pump is working appropriately
- Monitoring pump sites.

An example of follow-up documentation is given in Appendix 1.

A local or formal 'buddying scheme' is useful for further support and motivation. Social media has resulted in development of a number of informal channels for this.

Other considerations

Other aspects to incorporate in the service are listed below:

- *Ordering supplies and consumables*: a system to enable people to receive pump supplies and consumables may be established. General practitioners or family physicians should be informed if there are to be any variations in prescription items
- *Emergencies and technical difficulties*: insulin pump users and their carers should know when and how to contact their pump team and technical support for their pump. Pump users must have the provision to revert to subcutaneous insulin injections at all times in case of pump failure. This needs to be prescribed, kept when travelling and there should be clear guidance as to their use.
- *Information for other associated specialties*: it is helpful to have guidance on how to manage on pump therapy in hospital when the specialist pump team is not available. Linked specialties looking after people with diabetes who may not have a comprehensive understanding of pumps (such as cardiology, renal, ophthalmology and psychology) may benefit from education and healthcare professional support.
- *Information technology*: downloading pump data onto diabetes information systems is very helpful for identifying problem areas and to get more out of clinic reviews. Setting this up for your local clinic is important.

An introduction to continuous glucose monitoring

5

WHAT IS CONTINUOUS GLUCOSE MONITORING?

Continuous glucose monitoring (CGM) devices provide information about changes in glucose concentration in the interstitial fluid, which is present in subcutaneous tissue. Continuous glucose monitoring devices consist of a sensor (Fig. 5.1), which remains in the subcutaneous tissue, and a monitor, which connects either wirelessly, via a wireless transmitter attached to the sensor, or by a cable to the sensor. The monitor detects a signal from the sensor, which is then processed to give an estimate of tissue glucose concentration. The monitor may be a dedicated device, integrated into an insulin pump or running on another device (e.g. smartphone).

The sensor data need to be calibrated to capillary blood glucose typically one to two times per day depending on manufacturer to ensure accuracy. CGM sensors are typically indicated for 6-7 days, again depending on manufacturer. They measure the glucose concentration every 5 min. Continuous glucose monitors report interstitial glucose levels between around 2 and 22 mmol/L and values above or below this range cannot be reported. All systems use proprietary enzyme-based electrochemical methodology. These utliize an enzyme (usually glucose oxidase) that is linked to an electrode, producing a current proportional to the glucose concentration by a reduction-oxidation reaction at the electrode.

REAL-TIME VS RETROSPECTIVE CONTINUOUS GLUCOSE MONITORING

Continuous glucose monitoring devices can either record the glucose data, which can then be downloaded and reviewed later (this is called 'retrospective' or 'blinded' CGM) for diagnostic use with health professionals, or can display glucose information in real-time, allowing people with diabetes to detect changes in glucose and adjust their treatment as needed. The continuous glucose data provide information about the direction, rate of change, duration, frequency and potential causes of fluctuations in blood glucose levels. Retrospective CGM enables analysis of the trends of glucose concentration over a longer period of time in contrast to a capillary blood glucose monitoring, which only gives the glucose level at a single moment in time. Importantly, retrospective CGM is very easy to use, requiring no input from the patient during use. Capillary blood glucose values are required for calibration but this is done after the monitoring period, often by a healthcare professional.

45

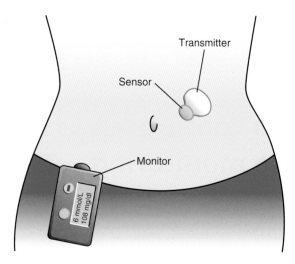

Figure 5.1 Continuous glucose sensor attached to transmitter inserted in the abdomen. This communicates to a monitor and can display real-time glucose.

An intermittent glucose monitoring system displays up to 8 hours of retrospective continuous glucose monitoring data, along with a trend arrow and a glucose value, on a handheld monitor when the monitor is waved close to a subcutaneous glucose sensor. In contrast to real-time CGM the intermittent CGM system does not provide alarms for high or low glucose. Stored retrospective data can be downloaded and visualised. The sensor is used for 14 days and is non-adjunctive, which means that the reported glucose values does not require verification with capillary blood glucose before diabetes treatment decisions are made.

IS INTERSTITIAL FLUID GLUCOSE THE SAME AS BLOOD GLUCOSE?

Glucose concentrations in the interstitial fluid are dependent on blood flow, metabolic rate and the rate of change of glucose concentration in the blood.

Trends in interstitial fluid glucose are representative of changes in blood glucose concentrations but peak glucose concentrations in interstitial fluid lag behind rises in blood glucose concentration by around 5–10 min. This is important when continuous glucose monitors are calibrated.

To ensure the continuous glucose monitor is as accurate as possible, calibrations should be done when the glucose concentration is as stable as possible. If there is a rapid change in glucose at the time of the calibration, there may be a large difference between blood and interstitial fluid glucose and this difference may be 'fixed' for all results given by the sensor until the next calibration.

Continuous glucose monitoring is not a replacement for capillary blood glucose monitoring in self-management of diabetes but may reduce the frequency of tests needed in some cases. They can be a very powerful tool for support and education.

WHEN CAN CONTINUOUS GLUCOSE MONITORING BE USED?

Continuous glucose monitoring devices are used in the assessment of glucose profiles in people with diabetes with consistent glucose problems on insulin therapy. The published literature on CGM shows that it has benefits in combination with intensive insulin therapy. After 6 months of continuous use of CGM, there is a reduction in HbA$_{1c}$, a marker of long-term diabetes control, which is associated with diabetes complications, such as blindness, kidney damage and nerve damage.

Continuous glucose monitoring is useful in guiding insulin adjustments for people with type 1 diabetes using multiple dose insulin injection regimens or insulin pump therapy and it may be useful in enhancing diabetes management and behaviour modification. It can help to identify and prevent unwanted periods f hypoglycaemia and hyperglycaemia and CGM can elp to reduce glucose variability (swinging glucose etween high and low).

WHO USES CONTINUOUS GLUCOSE MONITORING?

o gain benefit from CGM, people with diabetes will deally be motivated to participate in their diabetes are and, in particular, act on the results of the CGM. he monitors may be fitted by health professionals, eople with diabetes or their caregivers and people sing monitoring should try to ensure optimal calibra- ion. Sometimes, recording of events, such as meal- imes, exercise, alcohol, stress and hypoglycaemic ymptoms can be helpful.

There is very limited evidence to support the use of CGM in type 2 diabetes; therefore, CGM is mostly sed by people with type 1 diabetes.

ndications for CGM include:

- Continuous subcutaneous insulin infusion (insulin pump therapy). Continuous monitoring may be particularly useful in continuous subcutaneous insulin infusion where the ability to alter basal rates can be exploited
- Consistent disparity between capillary blood glucose self-monitoring results and HbA$_{1c}$
- Haemoglobinopathy affecting red cell life span
- Pre-pregnancy glucose optimization
- In pregnancy to optimize glycaemic control
- Impaired hypoglycaemia awareness (or hypoglycaemia unawareness)
- Poor glycaemic control, despite intensive treatment and appropriate self-management
- Suspected dawn phenomenon
- To evaluate the effect of a specific change in therapy

- In people who exercise to minimize hypoglycaemia
- In gastroparesis to support glucose management around mealtimes
- Suspected unrecognized hypoglycaemia, recurrent disabling hypoglycaemia or debilitating fear of hypoglycaemia.

Continuous glucose monitoring has also been used in people with normal glucose tolerance to provide additional information to usual investigation proto- cols in the investigation of insulin secreting tumours (insulinomas). It has also been used after gastric bypass surgery to assess risk of hypoglycaemia after meals.

There are no specific contraindications to CGM. However, continuous monitoring should not be under- taken in people undergoing continuous ambulatory peritoneal dialysis, as maltose (a disaccharide of two glucose molecules) used in the peritoneal dialysate is detected by the enzyme electrode.

GUIDELINES FOR CONTINUOUS GLUCOSE MONITORING USE

In the UK, the National Institute for Health and Care Excellence (NICE) Type 1 diabetes guidance (2015) recommends the use of CGM in adults with type 1 diabetes treated with pumps or multiple daily injec- tions (MDI) in the following settings:

- Commitment to use it at least 70% of time with required calibrations
- Despite optimized insulin therapy with pumps or MDI, experiencing either of:
- >1 episode a year of severe hypoglycaemia that has no obvious preventable cause
- Complete hypoglycaemia unawareness
- >2 episodes per week of asymptomatic hypoglycaemia leading to problems with daily activities
- Extreme fear of hypoglycaemia.

47

It also recommends that CGM should be provided by a centre with expertise in CGM use.

In the United States, The Endocrine Society guidance on CGM recommends real-time CGM in children and adolescents with type 1 diabetes in the following settings:

- HbA1c levels less than 53.0 mmol/L (7%) to reduce the risk of hypoglycaemia
- HbA1c levels greater than 53.0 mmol/L (7%) in those who can use the devices on an almost daily basis.
- No specific recommendations for children below or above the age of 8 are made in this guidance.

Intermittent CGM is recommended by the Endocrine Society guidance in paediatric and adult patients with type 1 diabetes for retrospective diagnostic especially in the following circumstances:

- Nocturnal hypoglycaemia
- Dawn phenomenon
- Post-prandial hyperglycaemia
- Hypoglycaemic unawareness
- Changes to diabetes regimen.

HOW TO CONNECT CONTINUOUS GLUCOSE MONITOR SENSORS

Sensors are usually inserted in the abdomen but other sites, such as the upper outer buttock or arm can be used (Fig. 5.1). When choosing where to insert the sensor, to ensure accuracy and reduce interference, the following is advised:

1. Locate 5 cm away from the umbilicus.
2. Locate 5 cm away from any recent sensor insertion sites.
3. Areas with stretch marks, scars, hardened tissue or lipohypertrophy should be avoided for sensor insertion.
4. Areas where there is the risk of chaffing from clothing, such as waistbands or where there is regular bending, should be avoided to reduce the risk of the sensor becoming dislodged or damaged, both of which can affect the quality of data collected.

It is also recommended that sensors are placed 5 cm away from an insulin pump infusion cannula and 7.5 m from a syringe or insulin pen injection site. Sensors may be a little painful when first inserted but are flexible and it is unusual to experience significant discomfort while using them. There is a very low risk of bleeding and infection.

Sensors are secured with dressings. Users need to be vigilant of any signs of skin infection, bleeding and to gauge whether the sensor is dislodged. Most sensors (and wireless transmitters) are water-resistant, so users are able to shower, bathe or swim while the continuous monitor is *in situ*. Deep sea diving while wearing continuous monitoring is not advised due to the impact of changes in pressure on the accuracy of data collection.

Types and uses of CGM are summarized in Table 5.1.

Table 5.1   Types and uses of continuous glucose monitoring (CGM)

	Retrospective	Real-time	Intermittent
Types of CGM	No display of sensor results. Data are downloaded at the end of period of monitoring.	Display of real-time glucose values, often accompanied by display of trends and alarm functions to warn of high or low glucose levels. Retrospective data can be downloaded.	Display of limited retrospective data, glucose value and trend arrow only when monitor activated. Retrospective data can be downloaded.
	Diagnostic	**Diagnostic / Therapeutic**	**Diagnostic / Limited therapeutic**
Purpose of CGM	To identify glucose trends and times of high or low glucose and adapt treatment as required.	This is ongoing use of sensing to complement intensive insulin therapy and allow the user to make real-time changes in response to glucose.	Diagnostic with partial therapeutic use as no alarms and limited real-time data.

FURTHER READING

NICE, 2015. Type 1 diabetes adults. (Draft for consultation, December 2014). Online. Available from: http://www.nice.org.uk/guidance/gid-cgwaver122/resources/type-1-diabetes-update-draft-guideline2.

Klonoff, D.C., et al., 2011. Continous Glucose Monitoring: An Endocrine Society Clinical Practice Guideline. J Clin Endcrinol Metab 96 (10), 2968–2979.

Making the best use of continuous glucose monitoring 6

Continuous glucose monitoring (CGM) is a powerful tool in self-management of diabetes and real-time technology can help people with type 1 diabetes to achieve a reduction in HbA_{1c} and /or reduced frequency and severity of hypoglycaemia. People with diabetes using real-time CGM are most likely to achieve these goals if they are able to wear a sensor continuously for at least for 70% of the time and if they have expert diabetes educational support.

To maximize the value of real-time CGM to people with diabetes, it is important to:
1. Ensure calibrations, where required, are done when glucose levels are likely to be stable.
2. Set personalized alarm thresholds and review them periodically to minimize alarm fatigue.
3. Use the trend arrow rather than the absolute value to make treatment decisions.
4. Remember that symptoms of hypo- and hyperglycaemia should never be ignored, regardless of the CGM date.

CALIBRATION

Rises in glucose after meals and at times when insulin levels may be low are seen in blood before they are seen in interstitial fluid. The delay is usually around 5–10 min though may be longer. When glucose is falling, the opposite may be true with lower glucose concentrations seen in interstitial fluid than in blood. Because of these differences between blood and interstitial fluid glucose, it is important to avoid calibrating CGM devices to capillary blood glucose results at times of rapid glucose change, e.g. following meals (Fig. 6.1). Calibrating may 'fix' the difference between blood and interstitial fluid for future reported sensor values until the next calibration, and CGM users should ideally calibrate when glucose is as stable as possible to optimize the accuracy of the sensor. This will often be first thing in the morning and before bed.

PERSONALIZED ALARMS

One of the biggest barriers to using real-time CGM on an ongoing basis is alarm fatigue. The monitors will alarm when the glucose is outside of set hypo- and hyperglycaemic thresholds and when the rate of change of glucose is very steep. The alarms can be frequent and disruptive, which means that they are switched off, ignored or CGM is stopped. Carefully setting alarms that suit the user and their desired glucose

51

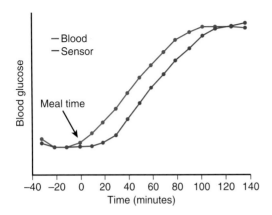

Figure 6.1 Differences between sensor (interstitial fluid) glucose and blood glucose following meals. Differences in glucose may also arise due to activity. To avoid errors from variation, calibration should always be performed in steady state (e.g. morning fasting and bed-time).

concentration window will help to ensure that alarms are more appropriate and less intrusive. Careful calibration of the sensor will ensure that the sensor signal is optimal and will maximize the likelihood of the alarms being correct, and expert support of self-management of hypo- and hyperglycaemia will empower the person using the device to take the appropriate action.

ALARM THRESHOLDS

Initial alarms may be set wide apart (e.g. at 3 mmol/L and 16 mmol/L) to minimize the frequency of alarms and may be moved closer to the target range gradually until the user is comfortable with the frequency of alarms and the glucose range between alarms. If hypoglycaemia is a frequent problem, the hypoglycaemia alarm threshold may be moved up to provide an earlier warning of impending hypoglycaemia and

allow for prevention. Over time, this may have an effect on hypoglycaemia awareness. If post-prandial hyperglycaemia is challenging, the hyperglycaemia alarm threshold may be reduced to provide earlier alarms, which may allow for an insulin correction bolus before significant hyperglycaemia occurs. Some CGM devices may allow different alarm thresholds to be set for different times. This can also help avoid alarm fatigue by minimizing alarms at desired times (e.g. at night).

ALARM SNOOZE FEATURES

The snooze feature on real-time continuous glucose monitors will notify the user if a high or low glucose state has not changed after a pre-set time. This means that the user can treat hypo- or hyperglycaemia but, if the carbohydrate or insulin correction was insufficient, the device will alarm after a pre-set time of minutes to hours. The snooze time can be personalized but should be lower for the hypoglycaemia alarm than for the hyperglycaemia alarm, as treatment of hypoglycaemia should take effect rapidly, while hyperglycaemia may take longer to reverse.

PREDICTIVE ALERTS

This feature warns the user if glucose levels are predicted to become low or high (predicted time alert) or if there is a sharp downward or upward trend for glucose (rate alert), so appropriate action can be taken before low or high targets are reached.

The prediction time and rate of change threshold can be manually programmed in some CGM devices. For example the prediction time can be set to 15 or 30 minutes. Based on the trajectory of the glucose, the CGM will then warn the user 15 or 30 minutes before it predicts the low or high levels (using the glucose value set in the alarm threshold). The rate of change threshold can also be programmed in some devices e.g.

).25 mmol/L/min or 4.5mg/dL/min. In this case the CGM will alarm if the rise or fall in glucose is greater than the rate of change threshold regardless of the absolute glucose value.

This is a useful feature. If set correctly, it can warn ahead of low or high sugars, and reduce delays due to lag time and time taken to treat hyperglycaemia or hypoglycaemia. However, incorrect settings can promote alarm fatigue. The settings (alarm thresholds, pre-set time programmes and rates) should be continually reviewed.

TREND ARROW

The absolute glucose value displayed on the continuous glucose monitor may be inaccurate, with values up to 15–20% different from capillary blood. It is also important to remember that capillary blood glucose monitoring devices may be up to 15% different from a reference laboratory glucose measurement. This means that the value displayed by CGM is a guide. However, the trend arrow, displaying the direction and velocity of glucose rate of change, is likely to be correct and provides the user with important information about how the glucose concentration is changing (Fig. 6.2). For example, if the glucose is 10.8 mmol/L 2 h after a meal but is falling, this may be the end of a mealtime peak and watching the glucose fall to target may be the appropriate action. However, if the glucose is 10.8 mmol/L 2 h after a meal and the trend arrow indicates a rapid increase in glucose, this may suggest an insufficient mealtime bolus, delayed absorption of

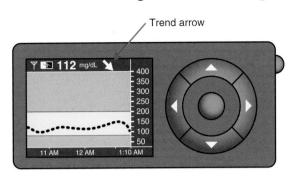

Figure 6.2 Trend arrow displaying direction and value of glucose change.

food or a problem with the insulin pump, and an additional bolus might be considered. In this scenario, the trend arrow informs the treatment decision and the absolute glucose value could be anywhere between 8 and 13 mmol/L.

SYMPTOMS

People with diabetes will often be familiar with how they feel during hypoglycaemia, hyperglycaemia and even during times of rapid glucose change. These symptoms are very important to maintain and should never be ignored, even if the CGM monitor suggests a normal or stable glucose. Diabetes technology can be inaccurate and may be incorrect, so it is very important to validate symptoms using a capillary glucose measurement.

Interpretation of continuous glucose monitoring recordings

7

Absolute values obtained from real-time continuous monitors should be confirmed using capillary blood glucose measurement prior to taking action, particularly to correct hypoglycaemia in the absence of symptoms.

Given the limited accuracy of continuous glucose monitors, particularly in the hypoglycaemic range, trends and glycaemic excursion data are key elements to extract from continuous glucose monitoring (CGM) and this information is best interpreted with diary information, including insulin administered, meals, exercise and hypoglycaemic symptoms. Analysis of retrospective monitoring should be performed with the person with diabetes and the impact of the monitoring period should be assessed in the clinic with consideration of repeated monitoring.

A STEP-BY-STEP APPROACH TO INTERPRETING CONTINUOUS GLUCOSE MONITORING

A step-wise approach to interpretation of CGM data is recommended (Box 7.1).

STEP 1 – BASIC INFORMATION

Who is the trace on, type of diabetes, treatment regimen, how many days was the sensor worn for, is

it a retrospective or real-time trace and what was the indication for CGM?

STEP 2 – ENSURE DATA ARE OF SUFFICIENT QUALITY TO INTERPRET

Most CGM software will provide different types of report with the data presented in differing ways. It is important to look at each report as they offer different information. Prior to interpreting CGM, the overall trace should be reviewed to ensure the information is robust enough to make treatment decisions. Missing sections of data, periods of time with rapid changes in glucose that do not correlate with the diary or symptoms and very straight lines should be interpreted with caution and periods of time where the sensor glucose is much higher or lower than the capillary values should also be reviewed critically. This information gives an overall view of the quality of the trace. For a sensor recording glucose every 5 min, there should be 288 values in a complete 24 h period; any fewer than this suggests missing data and it is important to identify where this occurs.

Some reports will also report the mean absolute difference as a percentage (MAD%), also sometimes called the 'mean absolute relative difference' (MARD). The MAD% gives an idea of sensor accuracy. In most

55

Box 7.1 Step-by-step approach to CGM interpretation

- Step 1 – Basic information on patient and CGM
- Step 2 – CGM data quality check
- Step 3 – CGM data summary
- Step 4 – Daily overlay view (trends)
- Step 5 – Detailed day-by-day view (patterns and behaviour)
- Step 6 – Masking for excursions.

studies, the MAD% for sensors is between 10% and 15%, suggesting that the sensor glucose is within 15% of the capillary blood glucose. For example, a reported sensor glucose of 10 mmol/L may represent a capillary blood glucose between 8.5 and 11.5 mmol/L. Some reports will also report a correlation coefficient or *r* value. This measures how tightly the sensor glucose tracks the blood glucose. A perfect 'straight-line' relationship between sensor and blood glucose will have a correlation coefficient of 1.0 but this does not mean that the two glucose values match perfectly, just that the relationship between the two is absolutely constant throughout the range of glucose. The sensor may be under- or over-reporting glucose and this may be amplified as glucose increases. As an extreme example, if the sensor glucose was always exactly double the capillary blood glucose, this would give a correlation coefficient of 1.0 but would clearly not be a helpful CGM trace.

STEP 3 – LOOK AT THE DATA SUMMARY

The next area to look at is the statistics summary. Reports include the number of glucose values, highest value, lowest value, mean sensor glucose, mean capillary blood glucose, standard deviation (SD) and the percentage of time spent in hypoglycaemia, target and hyperglycaemia. These values are usually given for each day and for the overall monitoring and, where needed, target ranges can be personalized. The highest and lowest values give the range of glucose but it should be remembered that all sensors have a low and high limit of detection and where the high or low sensor glucose range are the same as the limit of detection of the sensor, the actual glucose may have risen higher or fallen lower.

The mean sensor glucose is the average of all glucose values and the mean capillary blood glucose is the average of the calibration glucose results. These might be very different from each other depending on the glucose excursions seen in the CGM trace. The SD of the sensor glucose is a measure of spread of glucose values and is an indicator of glucose variability. The percentage time spent in hypoglycaemia, target and hyperglycaemia gives an idea of overall glucose patterns and may be a target for changes in treatment informed by CGM.

STEP 4 – DAILY OVERLAY VIEW

This view shows each day of the monitoring period drawn on top of each other (usually in different colours), showing patterns of glucose change over several days or weeks (also known as modal day view). This format is the most popular way of reviewing CGM traces and is used in illustrated examples for this book. Breaking this up into sections of the day will allow the identification of trends, for example times where there are frequent high or low glucose excursions and periods of the day where the same glucose changes occur.

Things to look for are: repeated hypoglycaemia, particularly overnight, after exercise and before meals; recurrent hyperglycaemia, particularly after meals; and patterns of downsloping or upsloping trends. Ignore outliers or extreme isolated hyperglycaemia or hypoglycaemia episodes, which are looked at later (Step 6).

Look specifically at: overnight, fasting, before and after meals, and during and after exercise, using the activity and food diary to support the timings. Remember to trace changes back, as glucose effects of alcohol and exercise in diabetes may occur several hours later or even the next day.

As a general rule, steep gradient downsloping trends reflect insulin action on glucose and steep gradient upsloping trends reflect food intake. Gradual downsloping may be related to activity, increased basal insulin or insulin taken with meal. Gradual upsloping may be due to inadequate basal insulin, stress or small snacks.

STEP 5 – DETAILED DAY-BY-DAY VIEW

This view allows each day to be viewed individually and each glucose excursion or event can be correlated with the diary and vice-versa, the glucose effects of specific activities or foods can be assessed. Longer-term changes, such as the difference between weekdays and

weekends; changes over the menstrual cycle; and changes during periods of stress, can also be viewed in this way. Reviewing this period can help with the assessment of patterns of hypoglycaemia, overnight glucose control, pre- and post-prandial glucose control, effects of correction doses, pattern of rebound hyperglycaemia, post-hypoglycaemia treatment and effects of lifestyle, exercise and stress.

STEP 6 – MASKING

Using a piece of paper, cover up the target glucose range on the daily overlay view, to show only the hypo- and hyperglycaemic excursions. This is useful to demonstrate the number and pattern of excursions very clearly and examine outliers or isolated highs and lows. Remember to trace excursions back to identify the cause.

Worked example 7.1: An example interpretation using this approach

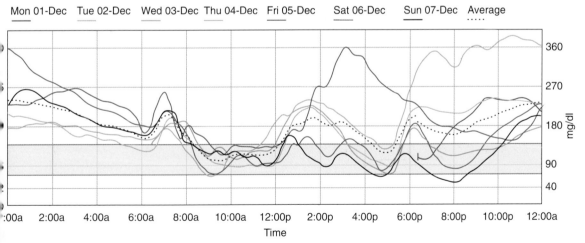

Name:	Mrs JS	**Correlation coefficient**	0.95
Diabetes:	Type 1 diabetes 1986		**Overnight:** Persistent downslope between 00:00 and 06:00 on most nights, falling around 5 mmol/L.
Treatment:	Multiple dose injection (MDI) regimen with once daily Levemir at night and aspart with meals. Carbohydrate counting.		**Before/after meals:** Fasting glucose above target requiring correction to target after breakfast. Borderline hypoglycaemia before evening meal. Using corrections.
Trace:	Retrospective		**Day-by-day:** Missed lunchtime bolus on Saturday 6 December.
Duration:	7 days		**Other events:** Delayed hypoglycaemia after exercise on Sunday 7 December.
Quality:	Good trace		**Actions:**
Number of values:	288 per day		1. Split basal insulin
Highest sensor glucose:	21.5 mmol/L		2. Review carbohydrate ratios as may change with alteration to basal insulin
Lowest sensor glucose:	2.9 mmol/L		3. Discuss effect of missing bolus with food
Mean sensor glucose:	9.9 mmol/L		4. Discuss strategies to avoid hypoglycaemia with exercise, including reducing aspart with the meal before exercise and using carbohydrate.
SD:	3.8 mmol/L		
% time in hypoglycaemia:	2		
% time in target:	61		
% time in hyperglycaemia:	37		
MAD%:	14		

In the following chapters we present illustrated cases utilizing real-time and retrospective CGM to highlight common clinical scenarios. We practise the step-by-step method to interpret CGM recordings in the daily overlay view, diagnose problems and suggest management.

Glucose profile in normal, well-controlled and suboptimal diabetes

8

The following chapter presents simple cases where you can practise using the approach outlined in Chapter 7 and make informed clinical decisions.

NORMAL GLUCOSE TOLERANCE

CGM in individuals without diabetes is mainly used in academic settings as part of research trials. However, it may be considered in those at high risk for diabetes or those being investigated for frequent hypoglycaemia. The normal trace below provides a useful reference point for glucose profiles in normal individuals.

Case: A 48-year-old woman of European origin with no history of diabetes. She has a body mass index (BMI) of 24 and a family history of late-onset type 2 diabetes in 1st-degree relatives. She does not report any symptoms and has an HbA$_{1c}$ of 5.2.

CGM RECORDING (Fig. 8.1)

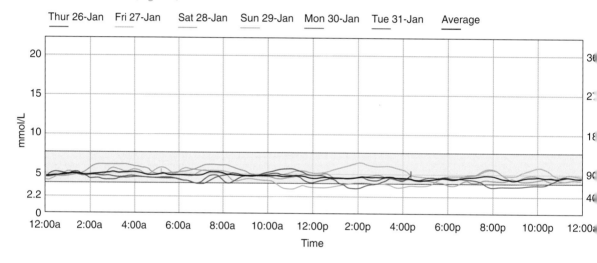

CGM DATA (Tables 8.1, 8.2)

Table 8.1	Average/total
Sensor values	1287
Highest	6.4
Lowest	3.2
Average	4.7
Standard deviation (SD)	0.7
Mean absolute difference as a percentage (MAD%)	5.2

Table 8.2	Average/total
High excursions	0
Low excursions	7
Duration above range	0
Duration in range	89%
Duration below range	11%
Valid calibrations	9

THE CGM RECORDING SHOWS

Adequate sensor recordings and calibrations were taken during the recording period. CGM data reflect a stable glucose profile with very little glycaemic variability (SD 0.7)

Overnight pattern displays no abnormalities with stable glucose levels throughout the night

Pre-meal and 2 h post-prandial glucose values are within normal limits, with no hyperglycaemic glucose levels

Brief periods of mild low glucose values are noted to occur during the day. These episodes are not in the fasting state. The low excursions (7) and duration below range (11%) reflect these mild drops in glucose levels with the lowest level being recorded a 3.2 mmol/L.

INTERPRETATION

CGM recording reflects very good glycaemic control and does not display any abnormalities requiring treatment

The low glucose values are unlikely to be significant. People with normal glucose tolerance can have glucose values as low as 3.5 mmol/L. The lower glucose range on a sensor is set up as below 3.9 mmol/L. Given CGM sensors' accuracy at the low glucose levels it is likely that the low readings detected are normal low glucose values rather than true hypoglycaemia. She did not report any symptoms, which is also in keeping with this.

MANAGEMENT

- No treatment required. Advise lifestyle modification if needed, to keep risk of future diabetes as low as possible
- Reactive post-prandial hypoglycaemia can be a very early manifestation of insulin resistance. The above CGM recording does not show any evidence of this. If suspected, a prolonged oral glucose tolerance can be performed. This can be managed with lifestyle modification (improved low glycaemic index diet, avoiding large meals, exercise and weight loss) to reduce the hypoglycaemia and risk of future diabetes.

WELL-CONTROLLED TYPE 1 DIABETES

Fine tuning well-controlled type 1 diabetes in the clinic can be difficult. Self-monitoring of blood glucose may not identify opportunities for improvement. CGM may reveal additional patterns that can be optimized to improve control whilst avoiding hypoglycaemia.

Case: A 27-year-old man with a 7-year history of type 1 diabetes managed on basal-bolus therapy with insulin glargine 14 units at night, insulin lispro 6 units breakfast, 4 units lunch and 6 units at dinner (ICR 1 unit:15 g). His HbA$_{1c}$ is 51.9 mmol/mol (6.9%). Home blood glucose monitoring reflected stable glucose readings mostly at 8–10 mmol/L (140–180 mg/dL).

CGM RECORDING (Fig. 8.2)

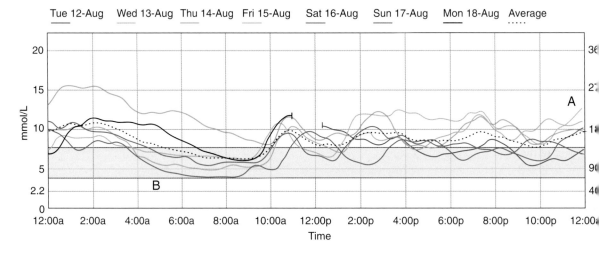

CGM DATA (Tables 8.3, 8.4)

Table 8.3	Average/total
Sensor values	1713
Highest	15.5
Lowest	3.9
Average	8.5
Standard deviation (SD)	2.2
Mean absolute difference as a percentage (MAD%)	14.5

Table 8.4	Average/total
High excursions	19
Low excursions	0
Duration above range	63%
Duration in range	37%
Duration below range	0
Valid calibrations	22

THE CGM RECORDING SHOWS

- Adequate sensor recordings and calibrations during the recording period
- The highest glucose recorded is 15.5 mmol/L and lowest glucose is 3.9 mmol/L
- Most of the time is spent slightly above the target glucose range
- Little time is spent below the range with no recorded hypoglycaemia
- Very stable profile with low glucose variability
- Consistent pattern revealing slight increase in glucose at bed-time (see A in Fig. 8.2), gradual reduction during night-time after 04:00 (see B in Fig. 8.2). Consistent glucose during the day but slightly above target after 14:00
- Good post-prandial control.

INTERPRETATION

- Good carbohydrate counting and bolus calculation
- Minor issues reflect basal profile of insulin glargine. Insulin glargine can have a slight peak (causing the low-gradient downward slope with gradual reduction of glucose during the night). This can limit its increase, which may result in day-time basal insulin concentrations being slightly low accounting for slight high glucose in afternoon onwards
- Insulin glargine may not have a full 24 h effect and can wear off before this period, accounting for high glucose at bed-time.

MANAGEMENT

- Good and stable glycaemic control
- If improvement in above is desired there may be several options worth trying:
  - Glargine can be taken in the morning to improve daytime glucose and avoid dips at night. Depending on the outcome, a slight increase in dinner aspart may be needed if bed-time glucose is high
  - Twice daily split basal could be considered with a higher dose during the day and lower at night.

SUBOPTIMAL TYPE 1 DIABETES GLUCOSE PROFILE

CGM can be a powerful educational and motivational tool to illustrate poor glucose control and the impact of behaviour on glucose levels. In such cases improved engagement, education and motivation is often needed to improve glucose control and CGM can provide a compelling visual representation of glucose levels.

Case: A 42-year-old woman with a 29-year history of type 1 diabetes is reviewed in the clinic. She is currently managed on basal-bolus insulin therapy with insulin detemir 10 units with breakfast, 8 units at night, insulin aspart 4 units at breakfast (06:00–08:00), 5 units at lunch (13:00–14:00) and 6 units (19:00–20:00) at dinner. She is currently experiencing significant problems with high glucose. She is physically active and is trained in carbohydrate counting.

Her HBA$_{1c}$ is 79.2 mmol/mol (9.4%). Home blood glucose monitoring reveals variable readings with poor consistency and significantly high glucose. CGM was done with a glucose, insulin and food diary to understand trends and help with further management.

CGM RECORDING (Fig. 8.3)

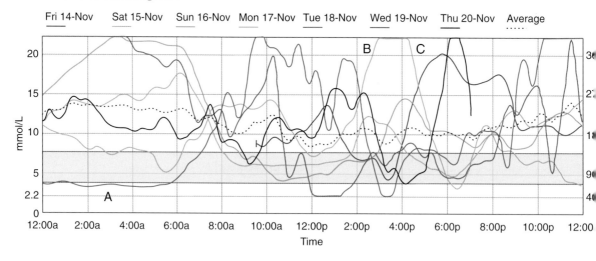

CGM DATA (Tables 8.5, 8.6)

Table 8.5	Average/total
Sensor values	1843
Highest	22.2
Lowest	2.2
Average	11.3
Standard deviation (SD)	5.4
Mean absolute difference as a percentage (MAD%)	11.4

Table 8.6	Average/total
High excursions	19
Low excursions	6
Duration above range	69%
Duration in range	25%
Duration below range	6%
Valid calibrations	24

THE CGM RECORDING SHOWS

- Adequate sensor recordings and calibrations during the recording period
- The highest glucose recorded is 22.2 mmol/L (CGM upper limit of detection) and lowest glucose is 2.2 mmol/L (CGM lower limit of detection)
- Most of the time is spent above the target glucose range
- Hyperglycaemia occurring at variable times preceded by multiple rapid upstrokes during the day in most cases
- Bed-time hypoglycaemia and one prolonged period of nocturnal hypoglycaemia (see A in Fig. 8.3).

INTERPRETATION

- Suboptimal glucose profile with large number of hyperglycaemic events throughout the day and persisting during the night
- The prolonged period of hypoglycaemia at night (see A in Fig. 8.3) is an anomaly and on further questioning, it followed a period of intense activity and omission of a bed-time snack
- The high-gradient upstrokes preceding hyperglycaemia suggest food (with insufficient or no bolus) as the most likely cause for hyperglycaemia. (Gradual upstrokes might suggest insufficient insulin but this is not seen.)
- Snacking between meals with no corresponding insulin bolus. This is confirmed on a food diary
- 'Pendulum swings' where some upstrokes have a marked downstroke following it (see B and C in Fig. 8.3). This could be due to a high dose bolus that is taken late (after meals). This will cause high post-prandial glucose (30–60 min after starting a meal). Once the insulin, which is given late, starts taking effect (peak at 60 min after injection), there is a decline in glucose
- On further questioning, boluses are frequently taken after meals, sometimes 15–20 min after finishing food
- Peaks are occurring at variable times, suggesting meal patterns are not at regular times.

MANAGEMENT

- Support and educate to more effectively. Match insulin and food, paying particular attention to bolus intake with snacks (or having carbohydrate free snacks) and taking bolus insulin before food
- Her high basal to bolus ratio is partially compensating for snacking. Her basal insulin may need reduction if her diet and insulin behaviours change
- Revision of diabetes-structured education and checking carbohydrate counting would be helpful. She may benefit from pump therapy but the above measures are recommended first.

Abnormalities of glucose profile at night 9

Frequent overnight testing can be very inconvenient for people with diabetes. CGM provides a convenient way to assess and improve overnight glycaemic control and often reveals issues not noted previously. This chapter demonstrates 2 common examples of abnormalities in glucose profile at night and discusses approaches to manage them.

NOCTURNAL HYPOGLYCAEMIA

Recurrent hypoglycaemia is unpleasant and has a significant impact on people with diabetes and their familie and carers. It can impact on activities of daily living, increases the risk of severe hypoglycaemia and can erod hypoglycaemia awareness over time. Often recurrent hypoglycaemia can be identified from self-monitoring bu CGM can be useful to identify the time, duration and magnitude of hypoglycaemia, as well as suggesting appro priate interventions.

Case: A 32-year-old European woman with an 18-year-history of type 1 diabetes is reviewed in the clinic She is currently taking a basal-bolus regimen with insulin detemir 24 units at night, aspart 6 units at breakfas (08:00), 4 units at lunch (13:00–14:00) and 8 units (19:00–20:00) at dinner. She is trained in carbohydrate count ing. Her carbohydrate to insulin ratio is 15 at all times. Her insulin sensitivity factor is 2.5 mmol/L. Her hom blood glucose monitoring shows high readings (12–15) in the mornings and she reports feeling very tired in th mornings. Her HbA$_{1c}$ is 49 mmol/mol (6.6%). CGM was arranged to investigate the discordance between HbA$_1$ and blood glucose values, as well as nocturnal glucose control.

CGM RECORDING (Fig. 9.1)

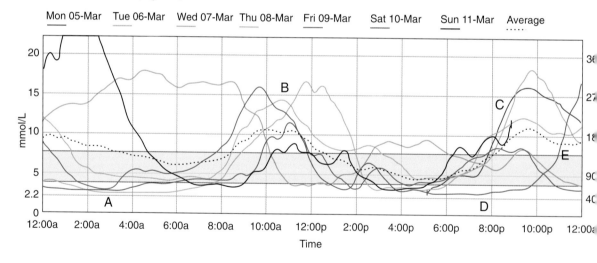

CGM DATA (Tables 9.1, 9.2)

Table 9.1	Average/total
Sensor values	1730
Highest	20.6
Lowest	2.2
Average	6.4
Standard deviation (SD)	3.9
Mean absolute difference as a percentage (MAD%)	9.1

Table 9.2	Average/total
High excursions	16
Low excursions	15
Duration above range	32%
Duration in range	36%
Duration below range	32%
Valid calibrations	13

THE CGM RECORDING SHOWS

- Adequate sensor recordings and calibrations during the recording period
- The highest glucose recorded is 20.6 mmol/L and lowest glucose is 2.6 mmol/L
- Most of the time is spent outside the target glucose range
- Prolonged periods of nocturnal hypoglycaemia (see A in Fig. 9.1)
- Hyperglycaemia following hypoglycaemic events (see B,C and E in Fig. 9.1)
- Pre- and post-breakfast glucose levels are mostly elevated (see B,C in Fig. 9.1)
- Post-dinner glucose levels are mostly elevated
- A prolonged period of day-time hypoglycaemia is recorded on Saturday. She reports having uncharacteristically fallen asleep between 18:00 and 20:00 in the evening (see D in Fig. 9.1).

INTERPRETATION

- There is reduced hypoglycaemia awareness overnight, with undetected periods of nocturnal hypoglycaemia reported by the sensor and one episode of prolonged hypoglycaemia during the day while asleep

- The CGM recordings demonstrate rebound hyperglycaemia in the evening, with glucose levels elevated after dinner following a low glucose pre-meal. This may be down to a reduced bolus with the evening meal to address the hypoglycaemia
- Her tiredness in the mornings is due to prolonged periods of nocturnal hypoglycaemia, which can affect brain function leading to fatigue
- The HbA_{1c} of 49 mmol/mol is within target, despite 32% of the time being spent above glucose range. The HbA_{1c} result is skewed as a result of the increased time spent in hypoglycaemia, which lowers the HbA_{1c} reading.

MANAGEMENT

- Hypoglycaemia awareness restoration can be challenging and should be addressed by education, support and by avoidance of hypoglycaemia under specialist supervision
- Her insulin detemir dose may be reduced and ideally would be split to be taken twice daily
- Her fitness to drive needs to be carefully reviewed
- Technology including real-time CGM with predictive alarms and insulin pump therapy may be appropriate.

69

DAWN EFFECT

The dawn effect is a hyperglycaemic excursion which occurs before waking and is not preceded by hypoglycaemia It is caused by counter-regulatory hormones, such as cortisol, growth hormone and adrenaline, being secreted prior to waking and is very difficult to manage with multiple-dose insulin injection regimens. An insulin pump can be effective in managing the dawn effect without causing hypoglycaemia by allowing increased insulin to be delivered during the early hours of the morning.

Case: A 38-year-old woman with type 1 diabetes and a 20-year history of type 1 diabetes. She is currently taking a basal-bolus regimen with insulin detemir 16 units at night, lispro 8 units at breakfast (08:00), 6 units at lunch (13:00–14:00) and 6 units (19:00–20:00) at dinner. She is trained in carbohydrate counting. Her insulin to carbohydrate ratio is 1 unit to 15 g carbohydrate except at breakfast, when it is 1 unit to 10 g. Her insulin sensitivity factor is 1 unit to 2.5 mmol/L. Her home blood glucose monitoring shows variable readings with highs before and after breakfast. Her HbA$_{1c}$ is 61.7 mmol/mol (7.8%). CGM was done to investigate her glucose profile further.

CGM RECORDING (Fig. 9.2)

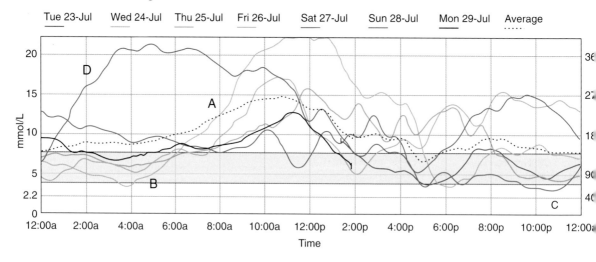

CGM DATA (Tables 9.3, 9.4)

Table 9.3	Average/total
Sensor values	1735
Highest	22.2
Lowest	3.1
Average	9.6
Standard deviation (SD)	4.7
Mean absolute difference as a percentage (MAD%)	9.3

Table 9.4	Average/total
High excursions	16
Low excursions	6
Duration above range	56
Duration in range	40
Duration below range	4
Valid calibrations	34

THE CGM RECORDING SHOWS

- Adequate sensor recordings and calibrations during the recording period
- The highest glucose recorded is 22.2 mmol/L and lowest glucose is 3.1 mmol/L
- Most of the time is spent above the target glucose range
- Little time is spent below the range, with six recorded episodes of hypoglycaemia
- Prolonged periods of hyperglycaemia starting at 05:00–07:00 and lasting till midday (see A in Fig. 9.2). Gradual increase in overnight glucose from 04:00 (see B in Fig. 9.2)
- Over-corrected hypoglycaemia at Saturday bed-time (see C in Fig. 9.2), with marked elevation of glucose on the following night (see D in Fig. 9.2).

INTERPRETATION

- 'Dawn phenomenon' with blood glucose rising from the early morning and increased insulin resistance at breakfast time

- Breakfast insulin not matching requirements
- Unable to increase night-time basal further as risk of overnight hypoglycaemia
- Hypoglycaemia management may need revision.

MANAGEMENT

- Revise management of hypoglycaemia
- Constant subcutaneous insulin infusion (insulin pump) would be indicated in this setting to improve overnight glucose profile due to 'dawn phenomenon'. Higher basal rates (30–40%) from around 04:00 would be advised
- Increase ICR at breakfast further to 1 unit to 8 g carbohydrate. With a pump, such calculations can be accommodated using the bolus calculator.

Abnormalities of glucose profile in relation to food 10

CGM can reveal useful information on dietary habits that may affect diabetes control. It also helps manage challenging situations in relation to food by providing an illustration of the blood glucose changes. In this chapter we present four scenarios and highlight how CGM can be used to improve control.

FREQUENT SNACKS AND BOLUS USE

Frequent snacks containing carbohydrate can give a 'sawtooth' appearance on CGM and can be challenging to manage as frequent rapid-acting insulin bolus doses can stack and increase the risk of hypoglycaemia. Insufficient insulin with snacks, however, may lead to hyperglycaemia. An understanding of insulin on-board can help to optimize glucose with snacks and some bolus advice calculators, especially those integrated into insulin pumps, will include insulin on-board in their calculations.

Case: A 19-year-old male university student with a 7-year history of type 1 diabetes is reviewed in the clinic. He is currently being managed with constant subcutaneous insulin infusion (insulin pump) and for the last 2 years has had problems with the dawn phenomenon. He does limited sports activity. He is trained in carbohydrate counting and is using the settings shown in Table 10.1. His HbA$_{1c}$ is 68.3 mmol/mol (8.4%). His blood glucose diary revealed high variation in his glucose readings. CGM was arranged to understand his glucose control further and recommend appropriate insulin adjustments.

Table 10.1

Time	Basal (unit/h)	
00:00–04:00	0.40	ISF: 1 unit: 2 mmol/L
04:00–09:00	0.90	ICR: 1 unit: 10 g
09:00–14:00	0.30	Average total basal: 11.6 units
14:00–00:00	0.40	Average total bolus: 32 units

CGM RECORDING (Fig. 10.1)

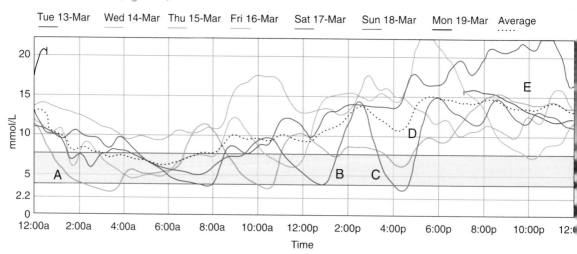

GM DATA (Tables 10.2, 10.3)

Table 10.2	Average/total
Sensor values	1507
Highest	22.2
Lowest	2.9
Average	10.9
Standard deviation (SD)	4.3
Mean absolute difference as a percentage (MAD%)	14.7

Table 10.3	Average/total
High excursions	15
Low excursions	4
Duration above range	73
Duration in range	24
Duration below range	3
Valid calibrations	10

HE CGM RECORDING SHOWS

Adequate sensor recordings and calibrations during the recording period

The highest glucose recorded is 22.9 mmol/L and lowest glucose is 2.9 mmol/L

SD of 4.3, suggesting high glycaemic variability

Most of the time is spent above the target glucose range

Occasional hypoglycaemic excursions (four in total and small duration spent in low range)

One episode of nocturnal hypoglycaemia proceeded by a moderate gradient prolonged downstroke, in-keeping with alcohol (see A in Fig. 10.1)

Frequent 'pendulum swings' with hyperglycaemia preceded by sharp upstroke suggesting food intake and sharp downstroke suggesting increased bolus use occurring at various times in the day including night (see B and C in Fig. 10.1)

Post-dinner glucose levels are mostly elevated (see D in Fig. 10.1).

Marked hyperglycaemia in the evenings after 18:00 with raised bed-time glucose levels (see E in Fig. 10.1).

NTERPRETATION

High glycaemic variability with snacking and delayed bolus use. This is responsible for the 'pendulum swings'. The delayed action of insulin on food results in hyperglycaemia with a delayed lowering of glucose

- ICR may be incorrect, especially in the evenings
- Frequent bolus use in the day has meant that he has reduced basal profiles, as some of the bolus insulin may have been stacking and working as a basal. Although this may be preventing hypoglycaemia, the basal profile should be re-assessed by basal testing
- Incorrect ICR, timing of insulin and basal leading to frequent hyperglycaemia in evening.

MANAGEMENT

- Revise carbohydrate counting, review insulin:carbohydrate ratios and support boluses at the time of snacks
- Pump download (to review frequency of boluses and timing in relation to food)
- Discuss avoidance of nocturnal hypoglycaemia after alcohol
- Basal rate testing and adjustment without influence of snacks
- Consider carbohydrate free snack options and ways to reduce frequency of snacking.

ALCOHOL

Alcohol prevents the release of glucose from the liver (hepatic gluconeogenesis) in the fasting state and increase the risk of hypoglycaemia, especially overnight following alcohol. Strategies to avoid hypoglycaemia after alcohol include reducing basal insulin doses, running a temporary basal rate overnight with insulin pump therapy and eating carbohydrate before bed.

Case: A 19-year-old male university student with type 1 diabetes, managed with basal bolus. On 14 units insulin glargine 14 units at night and carbohydrate counts with insulin lispro. (Typical doses 4 units breakfast 6 units lunch and dinner.) HbA$_{1c}$ 8.4%. CGM performed to assess glycaemic control further.

CGM RECORDING (Fig. 10.2)

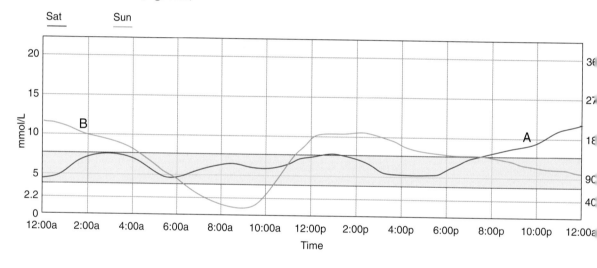

HE CGM RECORDING SHOWS

Went out with friends Saturday night when he had alcohol

Increased glucose Saturday night (see A in Fig. 10.2)

Downslope overnight with low glucose Sunday morning (see B in Fig. 10.2).

NTERPRETATION

See 'Alcohol' section in carbohydrate counting, p. 27

Alcohol beverages can contain carbohydrate, which causes an initial glucose rise

Alcohol can lower blood glucose by inhibiting hepatic glucose output, and low glucose early Sunday morning is a result of this.

MANAGEMENT

- Avoid bolus insulin doses with alcohol and corrective boluses after alcohol
- Carbohydrate containing meal or snack is advisable if moderate–heavy alcohol consumption
- Another option would be to take less insulin glargine (10% reduction) – however, ensure basal insulin is not forgotten
- On insulin pumps, temporary basal rate can be used to help with this (20% reduction over 4–6 h).

FASTING

Fasting may be necessary before medical procedures, may be undertaken for basal rate testing with insulin pum[?] therapy, or may be a personal choice and it is important to be able to manage periods with no calorie intak[?] Avoiding bolus insulin, careful monitoring and reductions in basal insulin may be required to maintain sa[?] glucose and CGM can be a useful adjunct to support fasting.

Case: A 32-year-old woman on insulin pump therapy for her type 1 diabetes of 20 years' duration. Insulin pump settings, as shown below. Good glycaemic control with HbA$_{1c}$ of 57.4 mmol/mol or 7.4%. Performs prolonged day-time fasts as basal tests. CGM readings during this period are shown in Table 10.4.

Table 10.4

Time	Basal (unit/h)	
00:00–04:00	0.45	ISF: 1 unit: 2 mmol/L
04:00–09:00	0.70	ICR: 1 unit:10 g
09:00–00:00	0.50	Average total basal 12.8 units
		Average total bolus: 32 units

CGM RECORDING (Fig. 10.3)

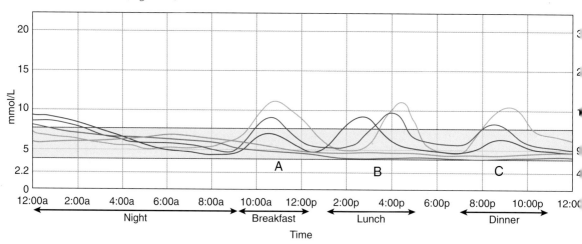

HE CGM RECORDING SHOWS

Stable glycaemic control during fasting and normal periods
No hypoglycaemia
Gradual downward slope overnight, which continues and persists until the evening
No rise and falls (humps) seen on fasting days (see labels A, B and C in Fig. 10.3).

NTERPRETATION

Basal profile seems very good, especially during day-time

- Overnight high and gradual drop – this could be due to insufficient bolus at dinner-time, with a slightly higher than needed basal rate.

MANAGEMENT

- Try an increased dinner bolus. If concerns regarding low glucose overnight, a slight basal reduction during the early night period (0.40 units/h from 00:00 to 04:00) may be needed.

RAMADAN

During Ramadan people fast between sunrise and sunset each day for a month. The change in timings of food, sleep and medications can significantly affect diabetes management with an increased risk of severe hypoglycaemia. CGM can be a very useful adjunct during Ramadan to support safe fasting, and strategies to maintain optimal glucose control include reduction in basal insulin during the day, splitting long-acting basal insulin dose and changing insulins to different formulations with a shorter duration of action.

Case: A 32-year-old man with a 22-year history of type 1 diabetes, manages his diabetes with an insulin pump, as detailed below. His control is good with HbA$_{1c}$ of 46.4 mmol/mol (6.4%); however, he does experience frequent hypoglycaemic events with good awareness. He is trained in carbohydrate counting (Table 10.5).

He is fasting during Ramadan in the UK, with the help of sensor-augmented pump therapy to avoid hypoglycaemia.

Sensor alerts:
- Low alert of 4.5 mmol/L or 80 mg/dL during the day and 3.5 mmol/L or 65 mg/dL at night
- Predictive alerts (rate alerts of 0.250 mmol/L per min or 4.5 mg/dL per min and 30 min prediction time)
- Low glucose suspend at 2.2 mmol/L or 40 mg/dL.

Table 10.5

Time	Basal (unit/h)	
00:00–03:00	0.45	ISF: 1 unit: 2.5 mmol/L
03:00–07:30	0.60	ICR: 1 unit: 8 g breakfast; 1 unit: 15 g other times
07:30–17:00	0.40	
17:00–20:00	0.30	Average total basal: 10.8 units
20:00–00:00	0.50	Average total bolus: 22 units

CGM RECORDING (Fig. 10.4)

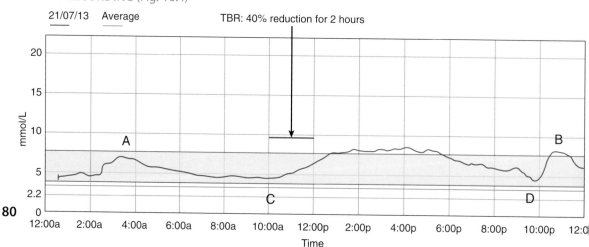

Fig. 10.4

Table 10.6	Average/total
Sensor values	281
Highest	8.3
Lowest	4.5
Average	6.3
Standard deviation (SD)	1.4
Mean absolute difference as a percentage (MAD%)	11.9

Table 10.7	Average/total
High excursions	2
Low excursions	0
Duration above range	24
Duration in range	76
Duration below range	0
Valid calibrations	7

HE CGM RECORDING SHOWS

Adequate sensor recordings and calibrations during the recording period

Highest glucose of 8.3, lowest 3.2, most duration spent within range with very low glycaemic variability

Good post-prandial control (see A,B in Fig. 10.4).

TERPRETATION

Stable control with fasting, which involves no food or drink from dawn to sunset (approximately 03:00–21:30 during the summer in the UK)

Meals taken at the times before dawn and after sunset. Carbohydrate ratio of 1:8 g carbohydrate was used for both meals

Gradual decline in blood glucose overnight

Temporary basal rate with 40% reduction used to ensure glucose does not go too low in the day with good effect (see C in Fig. 10.4)

Reduction in glucose before sunset possibly due to glycogen store depletion or increased activity (see D in Fig. 10.4)

- Increased ICR used at end of fast meal (same as for breakfast). Counter-regulatory hormones may be high at the time the fast is broken and may require increased insulin. Low GI foods and eating small portions is advised.

MANAGEMENT

- Reduce basal profile between 03:00 and 07:30. With a bolus taken at 1 unit: 8 g around 03:00 and possible disruption of circadian rhythm, there may be less of a dawn phenomenon. (Some people with type 1 diabetes using an insulin pump use a 'super-bolus' when eating heavy high GI meals that require a large bolus. The super-bolus is a large bolus followed by a reduction of basal rates for up to 4 h following the meal. This is because some of the insulin from the bolus will have an effect up to 4 h and will act like a basal.)
- Decrease basal 19:00–21:00 to avoid running low before sunset
- Fasting prolonged periods can be strenuous and difficult for those on insulin. Although it is advised that people with diabetes are exempt

from fasting during Ramadan, some may choose to fast. Stable control is important to minimize the increased hypoglycaemia risk. Hyperglycaemia is particularly hazardous, as during fasting people cannot drink and can become dehydrated

- The fast must be broken if there is hypoglycaemia or hyperglycaemia.

- Low alert: A higher value for the low glucose threshold (4.5 mmol/L in this case) during fasting is sensible, as it gives time for a temporary basal reduction to take effect (at least 60 min) since the intake of glucose to improve glucose levels is not possible during a fast. A lower rate at night prevents the sensor from alarming too frequently (which can result in alarm fatigue)

Abnormalities of glucose profile in relation to activity

11

Activity, both in the form of exercise and demanding work, is a frequent problem for people with diabetes. In this chapter we illustrate 2 examples and show how CGM can be used to optimize glycaemic control.

SHIFT WORK AND TYPE 1 DIABETES

Shift work is particularly challenging for people with diabetes with variable meal, sleep and medication times. It often leads to poor control in order to perform demanding shift work routines without the fear of hypoglycaemic events. Speed of absorption of food and insulin sensitivity can change over the course of the day. Self-managing diabetes and shift work, effectively and safely, requires frequent monitoring and an understanding of the effects of medications and food at different times. Insulin pump users can programme differing basal profiles for different shift patterns and CGM can be useful to identify real-time changes.

Case: A 29-year-old woman with a 14-year history of type 1 diabetes. She works as a nurse with regular shift work. She is currently being managed with constant subcutaneous insulin infusion (insulin pump) for the last 6 years and has had problems with hypoglycaemia during and following night shifts. She is trained in carbohydrate counting and is using the settings as shown in Table 11.1.

Her HbA$_{1c}$ is 45.4 mmol/mol (6.3%). CGM was done to understand her glucose patterns further, especially when on night shifts and to modify her insulin doses accordingly. She was on a night shift every night apart from Wednesday night.

Table 11.1

Time	Basal (unit/h)	
00:00–04:00	0.40	ISF: 1 unit: 2.5 mmol/L
04:00–09:00	0.70	ICR: 1 unit: 15 g
09:00–00:00	0.40	Average total basal: 12.3 units
		Average total bolus: 16 units

CGM RECORDING (Fig. 11.1)

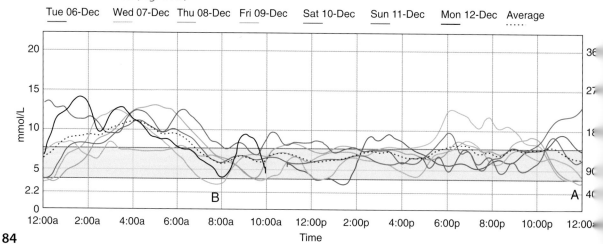

CGM DATA (Tables 11.2, 11.3)

Table 11.2	Average/total
Sensor values	1718
Highest	14.1
Lowest	3.1
Average	7.6
Standard deviation (SD)	2.3
Mean absolute difference as a percentage (MAD%)	14.2

Table 11.3	Average/total
High excursions	23
Low excursions	7
Duration above range	40
Duration in range	56
Duration below range	4
Valid calibrations	14

THE CGM RECORDING SHOWS

Adequate sensor recordings and calibrations during the recording period

The highest glucose recorded is 14.1 mmol/L and lowest glucose is 3.1 mmol/L

SD of 2.3, suggesting low glycaemic variability

Most of the time is spent in the target glucose range, a significant proportion above range and a very small proportion below range

The most striking feature is the flat day-time with reproducible stable glucose and the variability from activity and food noted overnight

Occasional hypoglycaemia (seven in total)

Two episodes of hypoglycaemia at start of night shift with a sharp downstroke, suggesting they may be occurring due to an increase in activity and in response to dinner bolus (see A in Fig. 11.1)

One episode of hypoglycaemia at the end of the night shift (see B in Fig. 11.1). This was preceded by an upstroke, hyperglycaemia and a moderate gradient prolonged downstroke. The gentle decline suggests it may be a combination of corrective bolus insulin, activity and reduced counter-regulatory responses overnight.

INTERPRETATION

- Overall very good glycaemic control with low glycaemic variability
- Flat glycaemic profile when meals not ingested, suggesting hypo- and hyperglycaemia mostly related to meals.

MANAGEMENT

- Glucose can be challenging to manage with shift work
- The above trace suggests satisfactory control; however, a trial of an increased ICR of 1 unit:12 g carbohydrate during the night may reduce the hyperglycaemic burden
- Avoid or reduce corrective doses of insulin if the last insulin dose given within 4 h. Using bolus calculator with active insulin time of 4 h will help.

EXERCISE

Different forms of exercise have different effects on blood sugar levels during the period of activity (see p. 2) Aerobic exercise usually results in a reduction in blood glucose whereas, counter intuitively, anaerobic exerc may cause a rise in blood glucose via hormones such as adrenaline. Activities combining both forms of exerc coupled with competition stress can have variable effects. Furthermore, the risk of hypoglycaemia follow aerobic exercise can persist for many hours and even into the next day. Insulin dose changes may need to co tinue well after the exercise is completed. It is also important to note that one episode of hypoglycaemia increa the risk of subsequent hypoglycaemia which may be further exacerbated by exercise. Reduced confidence performing exercise is a frequent problem in diabetes where activity should be encouraged given the benefic cardiovascular effects. CGM can be a very useful adjunct for people with diabetes who exercise frequently a can help achieve better control, performance and confidence in doing this.

Case: A 21-year-old man with type 1 diabetes on insulin pump therapy uses CGM. He regularly exercises (cycling and running) and competes at university and county level in the 400 m sprint. He exercises 5–6 times per week. His glycaemic control is stable with an HbA$_{1c}$ of 50.8 mmol/mol or 6.8%. His home blood glucose readings are satisfactory. He uses two different basal programs – normal basal and post-exercise basal for 24 h following exercise. His pump settings are as shown in Table 11.4.

At 2 h prior to exercise, he sets a temporary basal of 70% (30% reduction) until the duration of the exercise.

Table 11.4

Time	Basal (unit/h)	Post-exercise basal	
00:00–04:00	0.40	0.30	ISF: 1 unit: 4 mmol/L
04:00–09:00	0.90	0.65	ICR: 1 unit:15
09:00–12:00	0.50	0.40	
12:00–18:00	0.45	0.40	
18:00–00:00	0.60	0.50	

CGM RECORDING (Fig. 11.2)

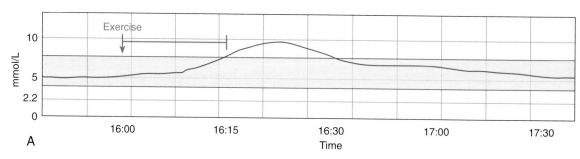

A

E CGM RECORDING SHOWS

A: Rise in glucose during and after a period of activity followed by gradual drop
B: A drop in glucose during a period of prolonged exercise
C: Stable glucose during exercise but gradual drop in glucose overnight.

TERPRETATION

e also p. 27 for Activity with pumps.)
Figure 11.2A demonstrates short duration intensive anaerobic exercise, which cause a rise in glucose.

This is typical for short burst activities, such as a 400 m sprint. The stress hormones released cause a rise in glucose despite increased consumption. A later period of drop in glucose can occur due to increased insulin sensitivity and as skeletal muscle glycogen is replaced.

Figure 11.2B demonstrates longer duration, moderate aerobic exercise where there is a gradual ongoing reduction in blood glucose, which continues after exercise resulting in hypoglycaemia.

Figure 11.2C demonstrates carbohydrate loading during exercise, which maintains glucose but a gradual decline and hypoglycaemia following exercise during the night recovery period.

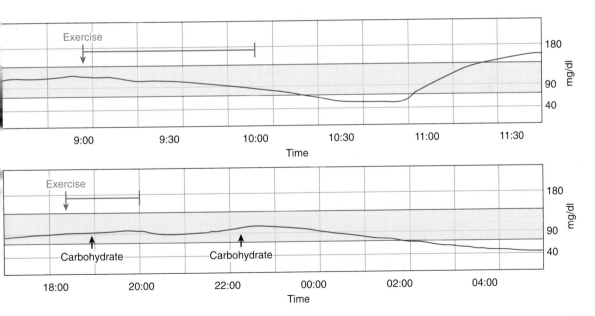

MANAGEMENT

- Competitive short duration exercise may not need an immediate reduction in insulin and may even require a corrective bolus after exercise. However, after exercise there is a risk of delayed hypoglycaemia which can be minimized with carbohydrate ingestion and insulin reduction

- Carbohydrate loading and reducing insulin befc predictable exercise are good strategies
- Reduction of basal insulin following exercise (ir this case a temporary basal rate of 60–80%) would be advised.

Using continuous glucose monitoring to manage difficult diabetes cases

12

is chapter discusses difficult cases and illustrates the application of CGM to improve glycaemic control.

HIGH GLYCAEMIC VARIABILITY

Glucose variability refers to increased swings in blood glucose. The importance of glucose variability and h
it is best measured is unclear but there are data to suggest that a high magnitude and frequency of glucose va
ations can cause vascular damage which may lead to complications, and can be difficult to manage. Gluc
variability is not reflected by the HbA1c, as the average glucose may not be suboptimal, and can be missed
blood glucose testing. CGM may identify increased glycaemic variability and, in conjunction with food, insu
and activity diaries can address reasons for this. The standard deviation of glucose is often reported from CC
traces and is the simplest method of assessing variability; a normal value is around 1.5 mmol/L (27 mg/dL).

Case: A 47-year-old man with a 29-year history of type 1 diabetes is reviewed in the clinic. He is currer
taking a basal-bolus regimen with insulin glargine 16 units at night, fixed doses of aspart 6 units at breakf
(10:00–12:00), 7 units at lunch (14:00–16:00) and 7 units (18:00–21:00) at dinner. He tries to follow a fixed c
plan. He works as a van driver with long unpredictable shifts, 7 days a week, brief periods of intense activ
and different mealtimes. He checks his glucose regularly in the morning, evenings and during the driving peric
which reveals occasional marked hyperglycaemia in the afternoon and very rare hypoglycaemia with preser
awareness. His HbA_{1c} is 62.8 mmol/mol (7.9%). CGM was arranged to support optimization of his gluc
self-management.

CGM RECORDING (Fig. 12.1)

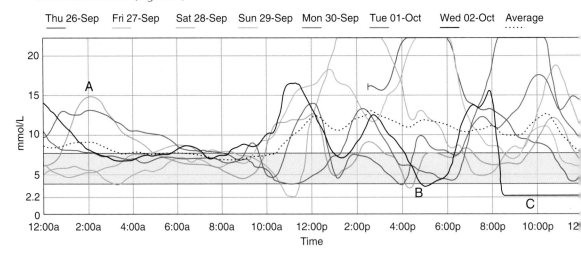

CGM DATA (Tables 12.1, 12.2)

Table 12.1	Average/total
Sensor values	1842
Highest	22.2
Lowest	2.2
Average	9.7
Standard deviation (SD)	4.8
Mean absolute difference as a percentage (MAD%)	13.3

Table 12.2	Average/total
High excursions	23
Low excursions	7
Duration above range	55
Duration in range	41
Duration below range	4
Valid calibrations	31

THE CGM RECORDING SHOWS

Adequate sensor recordings and calibrations during the recording period. Given high number of calibrations. Data missing from the first 14 hours of Thursday

Prolonged period of hypoglycaemia from just after 20:00 to midnight on Wednesday. Given loss of sensor data following this (and lack of correlation with diary), it is likely to be artefactual (see C in Fig. 12.1)

The highest glucose recorded is 22.2 mmol/L and lowest glucose is 2.2 mmol/L (upper and lower limits of CGM detection)

SD of 5.5, suggesting very high glycaemic variability

Most of the time is spent above the target glucose range

Stable glucose profile overnight apart from Saturday night

Frequent and marked hyperglycaemia during the day-time hours

Sharped upstroke with meals followed by hyperglycaemia

Occasional hypoglycaemia (seven in total and small duration spent in the low range).

INTERPRETATION

- Likely ate at 01:00 Saturday night (see A in Fig. 12.1). Otherwise overnight glucose control excellent (see A in Fig. 12.1)
- Mismatch between insulin and carbohydrate occurring frequently, leading to hyperglycaemia
- Recurrent 16:00 hypoglycaemia, (see B in Fig. 12.1). This may be due to mismatch between insulin and carbohydrate but may be exacerbated by physical activity
- Erratic activity and work patterns also resulting in increased variability.

MANAGEMENT

- Mismatch between insulin and carbs accounting for significant variability. Structured education to support carbohydrate counting would be very helpful to reduce this
- Revision of good driving practice and review of local licensing laws
- Increase dinner insulin dose to 8 units initially
- It may not always be possible to inject 15 min before lunch, given unpredictable nature and risk of forgetting meals; however, for breakfast and dinner this should be emphasized to reduce post-prandial hyperglycaemia.

IMPAIRED HYPOGLYCAEMIA AWARENESS

Severe hypoglycaemia, defined as 'hypoglycaemia requiring the assistance of another person to treat', may cau seizures, coma or death. Between 4% and 10% of deaths in people with type 1 diabetes are attributed hypoglycaemia. The risk of severe hypoglycaemia increases 6-fold in people with impaired hypoglycaemia awa ness. Such individuals do not have symptoms associated with hypoglycaemia and do not mount a counter-r ulatory response to hypoglycaemia which leaves them exposed to hypoglycaemia recurrently and for prolong periods. Hypoglycaemia awareness can be restored in some people by periods of complete hypoglycaemia avo ance. The use of CGM can be a useful adjunctive tool to identify impaired hypoglycaemia awareness. RT-CG with predictive alarms can also help to reduce hypoglycaemia in such cases.

Case: A 26-year-old woman, with a 23-year history of type 1 diabetes is reviewed in a pre-conception clin She has a BMI of 19. She is currently taking basal-bolus insulin with 8 units glargine at bed-time, 3 units asp at breakfast and lunch and 4 units at dinner. She is trained in carbohydrate counting and is using an ICR 1 unit to 20 g carbohydrate and ISF of 1 unit to 5 mmol/L. Her HbA$_{1c}$ is 41 mmol/mol (5.9%). She is havi frequent hypos and has had two severe hypoglycaemic events in the preceding 18 months. She is planning pregnancy and CGM was performed to investigate this further.

CGM RECORDING (Fig. 12.2)

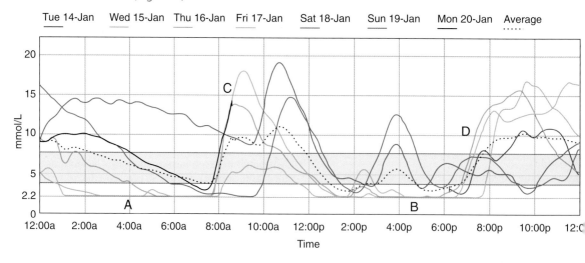

GM DATA (Tables 12.3, 12.4)

Table 12.3	Average/total
Sensor values	1613
Highest	19.2
Lowest	2.2
Average	6.8
Standard deviation (SD)	4.4
Mean absolute difference as a percentage (MAD%)	9.5

Table 12.4	Average/total
High excursions	15
Low excursions	16
Duration above range	36
Duration in range	28
Duration below range	36
Valid calibrations	16

HE CGM RECORDING SHOWS

Adequate sensor recordings and calibrations during the recording period

The highest glucose recorded is 19.2 mmol/L and lowest glucose is 2.2 mmol/L (lower limit of CGM)

Prolonged periods below range and above range

Prolonged periods of nocturnal and day-time hypoglycaemia (see A and B in Fig. 12.2), some up to 7 h

Post-prandial hyperglycaemia following hypoglycaemic events (see C and D in Fig. 12.2).

TERPRETATION

Significantly impaired hypoglycaemia awareness during waking and overnight with increased glycaemic variability

The CGM recordings demonstrate rebound hyperglycaemia, where glucose levels elevated after meals, which include an element of hypoglycaemia management

The HbA$_{1c}$ result of 49 mmol/mol is within target, despite 36% of the time being spent above glucose range. The HbA$_{1c}$ result is skewed as a result of the increased time spent in hypoglycaemia.

MANAGEMENT

- She is lean and very insulin-sensitive, making insulin dose adjustments very difficult in the setting of impaired hypoglycaemia awareness and increased risk of severe hypoglycaemia. Insulin pump therapy should be considered as it will allow smaller insulin dosage delivery and basal rates to be finely controlled to requirements
- Impaired hypoglycaemia awareness should be addressed with revision of hypoglycaemia prevention and management, frequent self-monitoring and consideration of avoidance of hypoglycaemia by increasing lower limit of glucose targets under specialist supervision
- She is at high risk of severe hypoglycaemia with considerable morbidity and even mortality. The use of real-time CGM with predictive alarms in addition to a multiple dose insulin regimen or insulin therapy may be considered
- Pregnancy should be delayed until her hypoglycaemia burden is reduced, she is established on an appropriate regimen and ideally with some restoration of her awareness.

93

PREGNANCY

During pregnancy, tight glucose control is very important to maintain maternal and fetal health and to redu the risks of adverse pregnancy outcomes. However, tight control is challenging in the context of dynamic chang to appetite, activity and insulin sensitivity. Insulin requirements during pregnancy increase over time and th may fall again late in the pregnancy as reproductive hormone concentrations change. CGM can help ident patterns and provide management strategies to reduce hypoglycaemia and hyperglycaemia.

Case: A 28-year-old woman, with a 14-year history of type 1 diabetes is 18 weeks into her first pregnan She is on a basal-bolus regimen with 32 units insulin detemir overnight and aspart 3 times a day with all meals. She carbohydrate counts (ICR 1 unit:10 g pre-pregnancy and currently 1 unit: 8 g). Her HbA$_{1c}$ 43.2 mmol/mol or 6.2%.

She is recording pre-meal, pre-bed-time, 1 h post-prandial and if symptomatic. Her glucose targets in pre nancy are fasting <5.5 mmol/L or 100 mg/dL and 1 h post-prandial glucose of <7.8 mmol/L or 140 mg/mL. S is having frequent post-prandial hyperglycaemia and hypoglycaemic events on home blood glucose monitorir CGM is performed to help improve her control.

CGM RECORDING (Fig. 12.3)

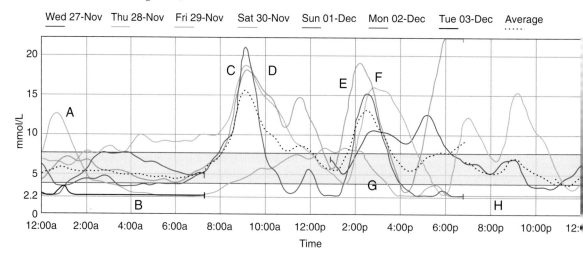

CGM DATA (Tables 12.5, 12.6)

Table 12.5	Average/total
Sensor values	1428
Highest	22.2
Lowest	2.2
Average	6.6
Standard deviation (SD)	4.3
Mean absolute difference as a percentage (MAD%)	29.9

Table 12.6	Average/total
High excursions	14
Low excursions	16
Duration above range	32
Duration in range	36
Duration below range	32
Valid calibrations	20

THE CGM RECORDING SHOWS

Adequate sensor recordings and calibrations during the recording period. Some data lost during the monitoring period which may limit some interpretation

The highest glucose recorded is 22.2 mmol/L (CGM upper limit) and lowest glucose is 2.2 mmol/L (CGM lower limit)

There is significant time spent above and below the target range

A large number of high and low excursions and marked glycaemic variability

Despite significant periods above and below the target range and large variability, her average glucose is 6.6 mmol/L, in keeping with good HbA$_{1c}$.

INTERPRETATION

She is aiming for a tight target of 1 h post-prandial blood glucose <7.8 mmol/L or 140 mg/mL

Significant periods of hypoglycaemia overnight and evening (see B and G in Fig. 12.3)

Some hypoglycaemic episodes occur after a steep downslope, suggesting insulin bolus (either corrective or for meal) as the likely cause (see A, B, G and H in Fig. 12.3).

Marked upstrokes (steep rises) preceding hyperglycaemia, suggesting rapid glucose increase after food intake as a cause for post-prandial

excursions (see C and E in Fig. 12.3). They occur at mealtimes (08:00–10:00 and 14:00–16:00). Mid-morning snacks around 11:00

- Marked downstrokes (large gradient downward slope) after hyperglycaemia suggest effect of delayed insulin bolus as cause for hypoglycaemia (see D and F in Fig. 12.3). This leads to marked 'pendulum swings' with periods of marked glycaemic variability.
- Due to physiological changes in pregnancy, peak glucose after meals may be sooner and the gradient of glucose excursions with food is steeper. It is more important to accurately match carbohydrates and insulin, and injecting bolus insulin before eating (if possible) is important.

MANAGEMENT

- An initial step could be to take a reduced insulin bolus (3–4 units) 15 min before meals and take the remainder of the bolus during or after the meal
- Split basal insulin detemir may reduce the frequency and severity of nocturnal hypoglycaemia
- Revise carbohydrate counting and explore low glycaemic index food swaps
- An insulin pump may address the challenges in managing her glucose during pregnancy. However a change in insulin delivery method may temporarily destabilize her glucose and the risks need to be discussed.

BARIATRIC SURGERY

Bariatric surgery has rapid and profound effects on glucose metabolism, even before weight loss and changes the way the macronutrients carbohydrate, protein and fat are handled. Insulin sensitivity increases and type diabetes often goes into remission but hypoglycaemia can become problematic in some people, particularly af gastric bypass surgery.

Case: A 58-year-old woman, with a history of type 2 diabetes and obesity. She had laparoscopic Roux-en gastric bypass surgery 2 years ago and remains on metformin 1 g twice daily. Recent HbA$_{1c}$ 5.5% (36 mm mol). She has symptoms of hypoglycaemia after meals.

CGM RECORDING (Fig. 12.4)

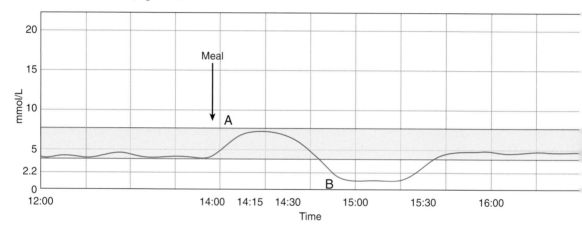

HE CGM RECORDING SHOWS

A normal fasting and before meal sensor glucose
A small initial rise in glucose (see A in Fig. 12.4)
A late episode of hypoglycaemia 1–3 h after food
(see B in Fig. 12.4).

ITERPRETATION

This is reactive hypoglycaemia
Reactive hypoglycaemia is common, is associated
with insulin resistant states and may be seen in
women with polycystic ovarian syndrome, in
people at high risk of type 2 diabetes, in impaired
glucose regulation and following bariatric (and
other upper GI) surgery
The mechanism is an insulin to carbohydrate
mismatch with excessive endogenous insulin
secreted in response to a carbohydrate load

- Reactive hypoglycaemia may be diagnosed using a
  prolonged oral glucose tolerance test or a mixed
  meal tolerance test that includes protein and
  fat. Very high levels of insulin and insulin
  c-peptide are seen in these tests, followed by
  hypoglycaemia.

MANAGEMENT

- Simple management includes changes to diet,
  aiming for lower glycaemic index foods and
  eating smaller meals more frequently
- Pharmacological management includes acarbose
  (which slows absorption of carbohydrate by
  inhibiting disaccharide breakdown), glucagon-like
  peptide 1 (GLP-1) receptor agonists, and in severe
  cases, diazoxide and somatostatin analogues have
  been used.

GASTROPARESIS

Gastroparesis leads to delayed gastric emptying. This can lead to initial hypoglycaemia followed by later hyp[...]
glycaemia following meals. It is often cyclical with periods of symptoms followed by periods of remissi[...]
Hyperglycaemia itself can exacerbate the symptoms. Therefore, a cycle can often occur of increasing hyperg[...]
caemia and worsening symptoms, which is difficult to break. Maintaining optimal blood glucose can reduce t[...]
frequency and severity of gastroparesis symptoms. Some studies suggest that the use of insulin pump thera[...]
has benefits in improving glucose profiles and gastroparesis.

Case: A 47-year-old man, with a history of type 1 diabetes, diagnosed at aged 13. He has had retinopat[...]
requiring laser treatment, has microalbuminuria and a stocking distribution sensory neuropathy to the mid-ca[...]
His recent HbA$_{1c}$ is 8.9% (74 mmol/mol). He has bloating after meals with nausea and occasional large volu[...]
vomiting.

CGM RECORDING (Fig. 12.5)

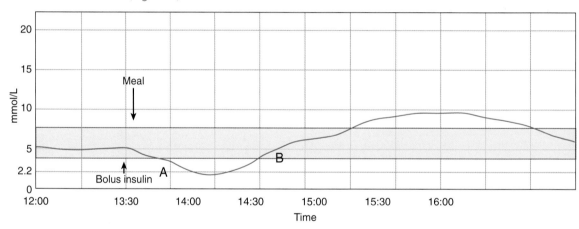

E CGM RECORDING SHOWS

A fasting and pre-meal sensor glucose in target
An initial fall in glucose after bolus insulin
(see A in Fig. 12.5)
Later prolonged hyperglycaemia (see B in
Fig. 12.5).

TERPRETATION

This is a typical pattern seen in gastroparesis
Gastroparesis is a component of autonomic
neuropathy and results from damage to the small
nerves, which run through the gastrointestinal
tract. This disrupts the waves of activity which
push food along (peristalsis), resulting in gastric
stasis, fullness, bloating, nausea, vomiting and,
sometimes, diarrhoea
Bolus insulin administered before meals is
absorbed within 10–15 min but food absorption
is delayed by gastroparesis. This means the
insulin initially causes hypoglycaemia followed
by later prolonged hyperglycaemia, as the food
is absorbed and the bolus insulin activity is
fading

MANAGEMENT

- Taking bolus insulin after food may be helpful
- Consider switching bolus insulin to a soluble
  insulin instead of a rapid acting analogue
- Draft NICE guidance for type 1 diabetes in adults
  recommends consideration of pump therapy for
  gastroparesis
- If using pump therapy, extended wave or
  combination boluses can help
- Consider pro-kinetic agents, (such as
  domperidone, metoclopramide or erythromycin)
  to improve gastric emptying.

Sensor-augmented pump therapy 13

This chapter demonstrates two case examples of continuous glucose monitoring (CGM) devices in conjunction with insulin pumps. The practical use and benefits of using real-time glucose values from CGM to influence insulin delivery via insulin pumps will be highlighted by these cases.

Sensor-augmented pump therapy is the simultaneous use of real-time continuous glucose monitoring with an insulin pump, usually with the continuous glucose sensor data wirelessly transmitted to the pump display. As with real-time CGM, an absolute interstitial fluid glucose concentration is reported, along with a trace of the preceding hours and a trend arrow. The sensor must be calibrated, ideally with a stable capillary blood glucose, as in real-time CGM use, and effective use of the data depends on support and diabetes education.

In its most basic form, the glucose sensor data are not utilized by the pump. Bolus calculations continue to require capillary blood glucose testing results and insulin infusion rates are not affected by the reported sensor glucose, even during hypo- or hyperglycaemia.

In more advanced systems, the system is able to switch off insulin infusion in response to hypoglycaemia or in advance of impending hypoglycaemia predicted by the glucose falling. The insulin infusion is suspended for either a fixed time (of up to 2 h) or until the glucose rises above a threshold. This ability to suspend insulin with impending hypoglycaemia reduces the magnitude and frequency of hypoglycaemia overnight. This linking of sensor data to insulin delivery is the first step towards a closed loop insulin delivery system (also sometimes known as an 'artificial pancreas').

Reviewing sensor augmented pump data combines supporting people using real-time CGM, reviewing CGM traces and reading pump downloads.

CASE 1

A 44-year-old woman, with a 6-year history of type 1 diabetes managed on insulin pump therapy for 2 yea following episodes of severe hypoglycaemia (see Fig. 13.1 and Tables 13.1, 13.2).

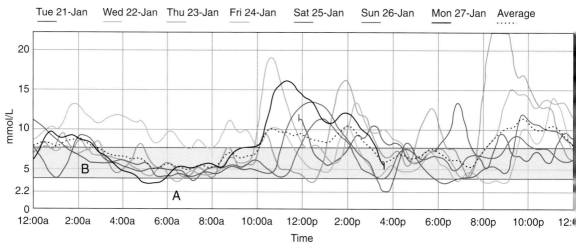

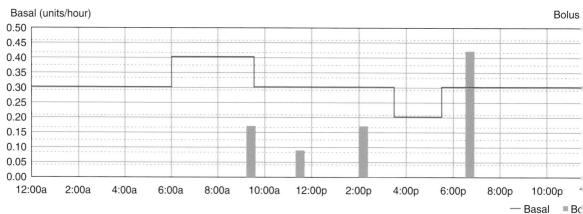

Table 13.1	Average/total
Sensor values	1744
Highest	22.2
Lowest	2.2
Average	7.8
Standard deviation (SD)	3.3
Mean absolute difference as a percentage (MAD%)	17.8

Table 13.2	Average/total
High excursions	28
Low excursions	9
Duration above range	41%
Duration in range	55%
Duration below range	4%
Valid calibrations	33

THE CGM RECORDING SHOWS

Adequate sensor recordings and calibrations during the recording period

The highest glucose recorded is 22.2 mmol/L and lowest glucose is 2.2 mmol/L

Most of the time is spent within the target glucose range

There are nine reported hypoglycaemic excursions. These occur in the early morning (05:00–07:00) (see A in Fig. 13.1) and in the afternoon and early evening

There is a downslope between midnight and 06:00 (see B in Fig. 13.1)

There is pronounced hyperglycaemia after some meals, particularly breakfast and evening meal.

INTERPRETATION

- Excess insulin overnight causing downslope
- High GI foods and insufficient insulin with some meals
- Insulin may be taken after eating.

MANAGEMENT

- Reduce insulin basal rate between midnight and 06:00
- Revise food diary and revise/refresh carbohydrate counting technique
- Adjust insulin:carbohydrate ratio with breakfast and evening meal
- Discuss importance of bolus insulin 15 minutes before meals.

CASE 2

A 32-year-old man, with 25 years of type 1 diabetes was managed on insulin pump therapy for 8 years as was unable to achieve target HbA$_{1c}$ with an intensified flexible insulin regimen (Fig. 13.2 and Tables 13.3, 13.

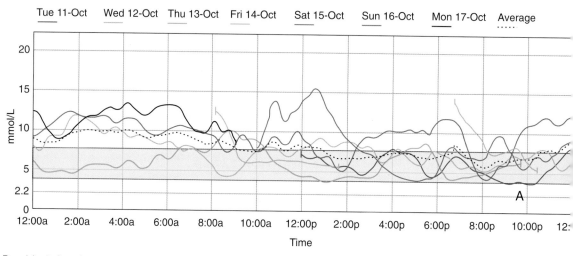

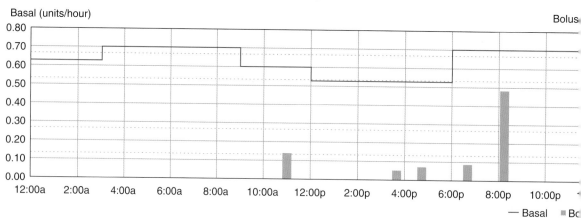

Table 13.3	Average/total
Sensor values	1371
Highest	15.5
Lowest	3.7
Average	8.0
Standard deviation (SD)	2.6
Mean absolute difference as a percentage (MAD%)	12.8

Table 13.4	Average/total
High excursions	20
Low excursions	2
Duration above range	47%
Duration in range	52%
Duration below range	1%
Valid calibrations	23

THE CGM RECORDING SHOWS

Some missed sensor data on Friday, with adequate calibrations during the recording period
The highest glucose recorded is 15.5 mmol/L and lowest glucose is 3.7 mmol/L
Most of the time is spent within the target glucose range
There are two reported hypoglycaemic excursions. These occur at the same time point in the evening of the first day of monitoring (see A in Fig. 13.2)
The sensor glucose is stable, but above target, overnight with an increase seen between 23:00 and 02:00
Post-meal glucose excursions are generally small.

INTERPRETATION

- May be eating late or eating low GI food in the evenings
- May be able to go to bed with a lower glucose without fear of nocturnal hypoglycaemia.

MANAGEMENT

- Revise food diary and review/refresh carbohydrate counting technique
- Discuss extended/square wave and dual/multi/combo boluses if eating low GI
- Consider increasing basal rates between 23:00 and 02:00.

Appendix

Insulin Pump Follow-Up Clinic

Date of appointment: _____

Patient details:

Pump details:

Insulin name:

Basal rates:

Time	MN	1am	2am	3am	4am	5am	6am	7am	8am	9am	10am	11am
Current rate												
New rate												
Time	MD	1pm	2pm	3pm	4pm	5pm	6pm	7pm	8pm	9pm	10pm	11pm
Current rate												
New rate												

Weight: B/P:

Current issues:

Blood glucose patterns	**Current**	**Changes**
Insulin sensitivity factor:	_____	_____
Correcting glucose levels above:	_____	_____
Correcting glucose levels to:	_____	_____
Target glucose levels:	_____	_____
Insulin to carbohydrate ratio	_____	_____
Total daily dose (TDD):	_____	_____
Basal: Bolus	_____	_____
HbA1c:	_____	_____
Frequency of set change:	_____	_____
Frequency of cannula change:	_____	_____
Name of infusion set:	_____	_____
Home blood glucose (min. 4-6 day):	Yes/No	
Injection sites inspected:	Yes/No	
Set change observed:	Yes/No	

Trouble shooting

Discussed guidelines on low glucose levels:	Yes/No
Discussed guidelines on high glucose levels:	Yes/No
Discussed preventing diabetic ketoacidosis:	Yes/No
Discussed guidelines for sick days:	Yes/No
Discussed how to respond to a pump alarm:	Yes/No
Discussed action plan for switching back to conventional injections:	Yes/No

107

Appendix 1 Example of follow-up documentation for use in clinic reviews. (MN = midnight, MD = midday)

Check the patient can carry out the following:

Suspending the pump:	Yes/No
Setting a single and multiple basal rate:	Yes/No
Setting a temporary basal rate:	Yes/No
Carrying out a self test:	Yes/No
Reviewing the alarm history:	Yes/No
Clearing an alarm:	Yes/No
Adjusting the maximum basal and bolus screen:	Yes/No
Bolus wizard/advisor:	Yes/No

Ensure the patient has the following contact numbers:

Diabetes nurse:	Yes/No
Diabetes dietician:	Yes/No
Insulin pump representative contact:	Yes/No
Insulin pump company customer services number:	Yes/No
Insulin pump company 24-hour helpline:	Yes/No

Plan:

Appendix 1 *(Continued)*

Index